The Theory of ADVANCED FIRST AID

The Theory of ADVANCED FIRST AID

by

J.A. Wood

MB, BS, MRCS, LRCP, MRCGP, DObst RCOG

Deputy Branch Medical Officer

Leicestershire Branch of the

British Red Cross Society

SPRINGER SCIENCE+BUSINESS MEDIA, LLC

Published in the UK and Europe by
MTP Press Limited
Falcon House
Lancaster, England

British Library Cataloguing in Publication Data
Wood, J.A.
The theory of advanced first aid.
1. First aid in illness and injury
I. Title
616.02'52 RC86.7

ISBN 978-0-85200-989-5

Published in the USA by
MTP Press

Library of Congress Cataloging-in-publication Data

Wood, J.A.
The theory of advanced first aid.
Includes index.
1. First aid in illness and injury. 2. Medical emergencies. I. Title
[DNLM: 1. First Aid. WA 292 W876t]
RC86.7.W66 1985 616.02'52 85-23901

ISBN 978-0-85200-989-5 ISBN 978-94-017-3513-1 (eBook)
DOI 10.1007/978-94-017-3513-1

Photoset by David John (Services) Ltd., Maidenhead, Berks.

Contents

Preface

When someone has successfully completed a Standard First Aid Course, they often have a desire to extend their knowledge of first aid. Thc aim of this book is to give the holders of a Standard First Aid Certificate the opportunity to study the principles of first aid in greater detail. It is not intended to convert the first aider into a highly trained paramedic – so a discussion on the use of intravenous fluids, defibrillators etc., is beyond the scope of this book.

It is hoped that the book will provide a useful in-depth study for demonstrators, instructors and first aiders likely to be involved in ambulance duties.

I am very grateful to Brigadier D.D. O'Brien, Chief Medical Adviser, British Red Cross Society and Mrs. R.H. Smith, Assistant Branch Director (Training), Leicestershire Branch of the British Red Cross Society for their helpful comments and encouragement.

I acknowledge the use of illustrations from the Clinical Symposia Series by CIBA on the "Heimlich Manoeuvre" to form the basis of Figures 3.7, 3.8 and 3.9.

Foreword

Standard first aid books tend to concentrate on practical descriptions of what to do in an emergency with the minimum of simple anatomy, physiology and pathology consistent with "the need to know."

Dr. John Wood, who has considerable experience as a lecturer in first aid with the British Red Cross, has recognised a desire amongst the more expert of first aiders to learn something more of the background of why we do some procedures and this book is intended to meet that need. It is written in simple terms and there is a useful glossary of words used with which the layman may not be familiar. First aiders will also welcome the section on medical conditions which they may encounter. In essence, it is a study, in a little more depth, of the rationale of standard first aid, without straying into the more advanced technical field of the paramedic. It does not repeat details of procedures which are adequately described in standard first aid texts and should be used, not to supplant, but to complement the latter.

D. Declan O'Brien,
Chief Medical Adviser,
British Red Cross Society

1
The skeleton

THE STRUCTURE AND RESPONSE TO INJURY

The main supporting structure of the body is an internal skeleton of bone. It also protects the soft, delicate tissues of the internal organs and, with bones acting as levers, allows movement by the action of muscles across joints. The inside of some bones contains marrow, which is an important source of blood cells.

Certain parts of the skeleton have obvious protective functions – the skull and chest wall.

There are three types of bone:

(1) long bones,
(2) short bones,
(3) flat bones.

Long bones are found in the limbs and consist of a shaft and two ends. The central cavity of the shaft contains bone marrow. The bone is covered by a tough layer of tissue called the periosteum, which nourishes the underlying bone through its blood vessels, and is capable of forming fresh bone if the long bone is injured.

Short bones occur where strength and compactness are required with limited movement. A number of short bones form the construction of the wrist and foot.

Flat bones are used where delicate structures require protection – such as the skull protecting the brain, and where a broad surface is required to provide for the attachment of several powerful muscles (as in the shoulder and pelvic girdles).

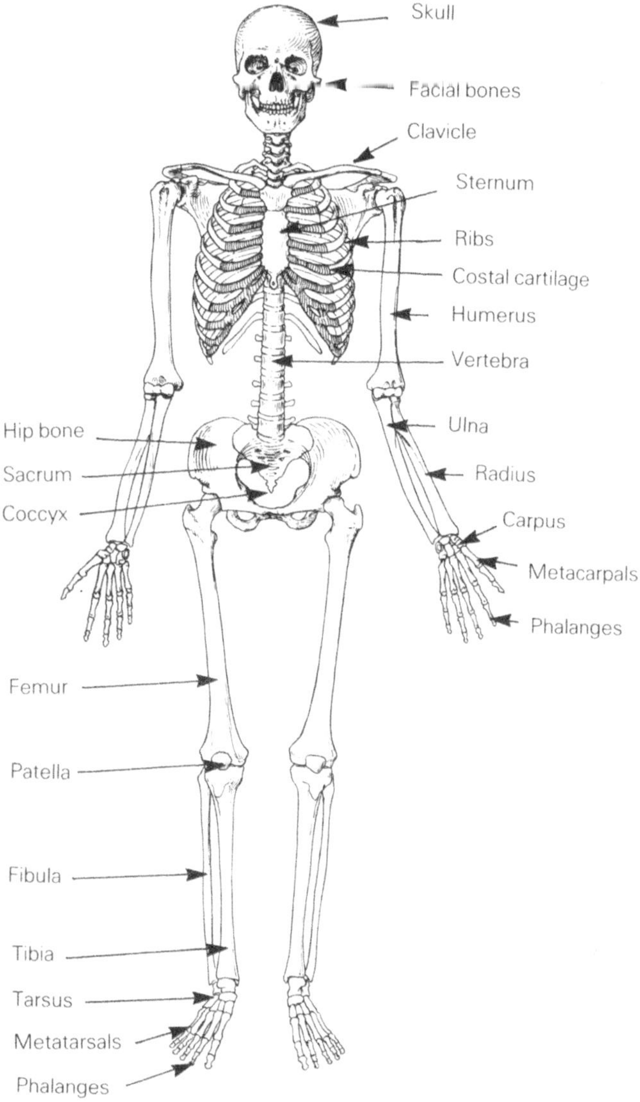

Figure 1.1 The skeletal system

The skeleton (Figure 1.1) is divided into:

(1) the bones of the head,
(2) the bones of the trunk,
(3) the bones of the upper limb,
(4) the bones of the lower limb.

The bones of the head

(1) The skull,
(2) The facial bones.

The skull

The skull is made up of a large number of flat bones, which form a cavity to contain and protect the brain. The bones are joined together so closely that no movement is possible between them. The base of the skull contains a large opening where the spinal cord passes from the skull into the vertebral column.

The facial bones

The upper part of the facial structure is fixed to the skull, and forms the structure of the face, with cavities for the eyes, nose and mouth.

The lower part of the facial structure is the jaw, or mandible, which is freely movable. It holds the lower set of teeth.

The bones of the trunk

(1) The breast bone, or sternum,
(2) The ribs,
(3) The vertebral column.

The sternum

The sternum is situated at the front of the chest and is a flat, oblong bone, shaped rather like a broad dagger. It gives protection to the heart and the large blood vessels. The inside of the sternum is a highly vascular spongy structure, with red marrow filling the spaces. The clavicles join the sternum at its upper end and seven pairs of ribs are attached to the sternum through costal cartilages.

The ribs

There are 12 pairs of ribs. Each is a flat bone in the shape of an arch, running from the vertebral column at the back, to the sternum at the front. They form the side walls of the chest, protecting the major organs in the chest and are capable of movement during breathing.

The ribs are divided into true ribs, false ribs and floating ribs.

The seven pairs of *true ribs* are joined directly to the sternum by costal cartilages.

The five pairs of *false ribs* are joined indirectly to the sternum – their cartilages are joined to the cartilage of the rib above.

The two pairs of *floating ribs* are joined to the vertebral column at the back, but at the front they are not joined to either the sternum or the rib above.

The vertebral column

The central axis of the body is the vertebral column, which supports the weight of the trunk and gives protection to the spinal cord. It consists of 33 bones called vertebrae. They are separated by thick pads of cartilage called intervertebral discs.

Although there is limited movement between each vertebra, the whole vertebral column allows considerable range of movement of the trunk, giving flexibility to the body.

The vertebrae are divided into groups according to the position they occupy: seven cervical (neck), 12 thoracic (chest), five lumbar (back), five sacral and four coccygeal (pelvis).

The cervical vertebrae are small and curve forward slightly as a group. The first vertebra, the atlas, has special sockets which articulate with the base of the skull and allow a nodding action of the head. The second cervical vertebra, the axis, allows a horizontal turning movement to the head.

The thoracic vertebrae each have a rib attached to them.

The lumbar vertebrae are large. Several powerful muscles are attached to them to hold the trunk upright in the standing position.

The sacral vertebrae are fused together, forming the sacrum.

The coccygeal vertebrae are also fused together, forming the coccyx – which represents the bones forming the animal tail.

The intervertebral discs act as cushions between each vertebra and help to neutralize the shocks to the spine and brain produced by jumping onto the feet.

Bones of the upper limb

(1) The clavicle, or collar bone, } the shoulder girdle
(2) The scapula or shoulder blade, }
(3) The humerus,
(4) The radius, } the forearm
(5) The ulna, }
(6) The carpus,
(7) The metacarpals,
(8) The phalanges.

The clavicle

This bone lies horizontally at the base of the neck and is easily felt just under the skin. It enables the arm to swing clear of the trunk by bracing the shoulder backwards. It is easily and frequently fractured by indirect force – a fall on the outstretched hand. The weight of the arm pulls on the outer part of the fractured clavicle, dragging it down and giving the characteristic deformity to the clavicle.

The scapula

The scapula is a large, flat, triangular bone which lies over the ribs at the back of the chest. It has several muscles attached to it and these give a wide range of movement to the shoulder. They also give some protection to the scapula, which is therefore not often fractured. The outer angle forms a cavity to articulate with the humerus at the shoulder joint.

The humerus

This is the longest bone in the upper limb. Several large muscles are associated with it and, at its lower end, it articulates with the radius and ulna to form the elbow joint.

The radius

The radius is the bone on the outer part of the forearm.

The ulna

This is the bone on the inside of the forearm.

The carpus

The carpus, or wrist, consists of eight short bones arranged in two rows of four bones. They glide on one another to give some movement at the wrist.

The metacarpal bones

These are miniature long bones that run across the palm of the hand. The metacarpals which articulate with the fingers run almost parallel with one another, and the prominence of the knuckles is formed by the heads of the metacarpal bones. The metacarpal articulating with the thumb has been rotated 90° through its long axis. This allows the thumb to move across the palm and increases the power of the grip when the fingers and thumb are bent.

The phalanges

The phalanges are small long bones forming the fingers and thumb. There are 14 bones – three for each finger and two for the thumb.

Bones of the lower limb

(1) The hip bone,
(2) The femur,
(3) The patella,
(4) The tibia,
(5) The fibula,
(6) The tarsus,

(7) The metatarsals,
(8) The phalanges.

The hip bone

The hip bone forms one half of the pelvis. It is joined, in the front, to the opposite hip bone, and to the sacrum at the back. This complete assembly of bones forms the pelvic girdle (Figure 1.2). The upper part of the hip bone, the crest, can be felt under the skin on the side of the pelvis, and forms the lower limit of the waist.

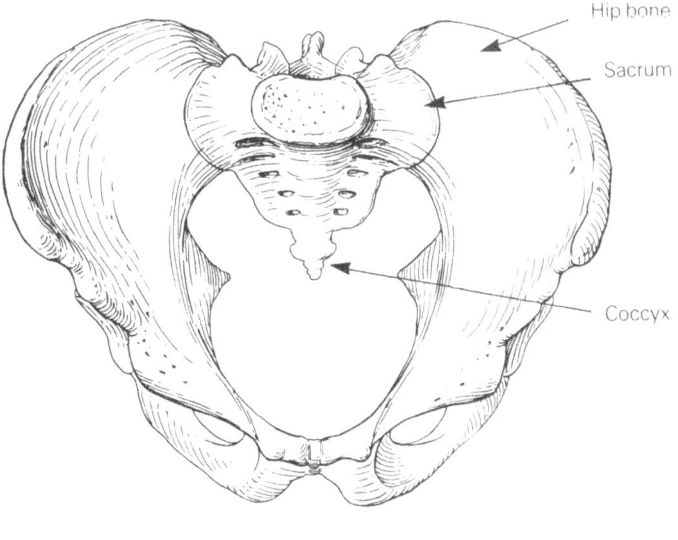

Figure 1.2 The pelvis

The femur

This is a long bone which slopes inwards from the hip towards the knee. It is the strongest bone in the body. The upper end has a round head which articulates with the acetabulum in the hip bone, forming the hip joint. The head of the femur is joined to the shaft by the neck. The lower end has two surfaces to articulate with the tibia at the knee joint.

The femur is frequently the site of a fracture. An indirect force is usually involved – when the casualty trips over. The trunk continues to move forward and the casualty loses balance. Over the age of 60, a fracture of the femur is a common result owing to degenerative changes due to age, which have weakened that part of the bone.

The patella

The patella is a triangular bone situated in front of the knee joint. It lies in the tendon of the quadriceps muscle (from the thigh to the tibia).

The tibia

This is a long bone situated on the inside of the leg, from the knee to the ankle. Attached to it are several muscles controlling movement in the ankle and foot.

The fibula

This is a long bone alongside the tibia, on the outer side of the leg. It is a slender bone, which does not form part of the knee joint and does not carry body weight.

The lower ends of the tibia and fibula articulate with the ankle. They are also connected to the foot by strong ligaments. These are frequently damaged when extra stress is put on the joint.

The tarsus

This consists of seven short bones which make up the back of the foot.

The metatarsals

These are miniature long bones between the tarsal bones and the phalanges.

The phalanges

The phalanges of the feet correspond with the phalanges of the hand. They are smaller but number 14 – three for each toe, apart from the big toe, which has two.

The foot forms a right angle with the leg. The tarsal and metatarsal bones are arranged so that they form an arch along and across the foot. The result of this is that the weight of the body is not transmitted directly through the tarsal bones, but is spread through the tarsal and metatarsal bones to the phalanges.

REPAIR OF BONE DAMAGE

When a bone is injured, it often results in a fracture. If the conditions are satisfactory, the repair process is started almost immediately and continues until the repair is complete.

The healing process occurs in five stages (Figure 1.3):

(1) haematoma formation,
(2) subperiosteal cell growth,
(3) callus formation,
(4) consolidation,
(5) remodelling.

Haematoma formation

Blood vessels are usually damaged as a result of the same force which produced the fracture. The collection of blood (haematoma) may lift up the periosteum layer covering the bone.

Subperiosteal cell growth

Within a very short time, cells from beneath the raised periosteum enter the haematoma and gradually transform it into a healing tissue (granulation tissue).

Callus formation

Bone cells in the granulation tissue lay down immature bone on bridging fibres (collagen) to form 'woven bone'. This callus formation may be felt at the site of a fracture.

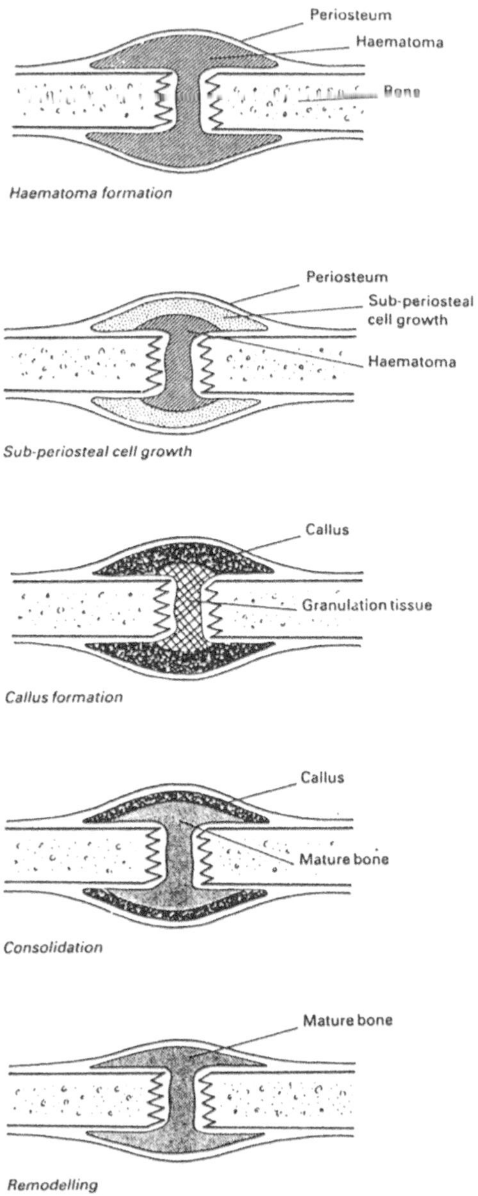

Figure 1.3 Repair of bone damage

Consolidation

The woven bone is gradually replaced by mature bone.

Remodelling

Excess callus bone is removed and the bone assumes its normal shape. The ability to remodel after a fracture is greatest in children and it can be so effective that the site of fracture may be indistinguishable on an X-ray. Fractures in adults usually leave some mark on the bone.

2
The skin

The entire surface of the body is covered by skin, which protects the tissue framework of the body. It also turns in to line the various openings in the body: mouth, nostrils, ear canal, anus and vagina.

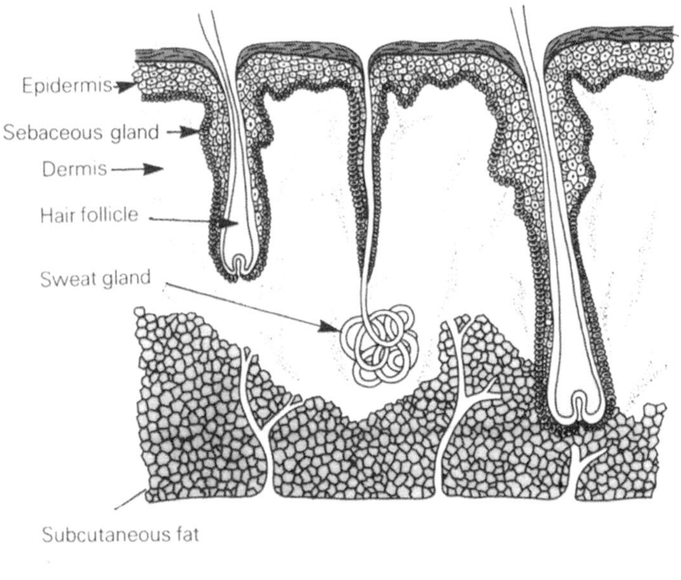

Figure 2.1 The structure of skin

It consists of two layers, the epidermis and dermis (Figure 2.1). Underneath these layers is a layer of subcutaneous fat.

The epidermis

This consists of several layers of cells which are continually being worn away by friction. The actual number of layers varies with the amount of friction the skin has to withstand. The epidermis is thickest on the palm of the hand and sole of the foot – and very thin between the fingers and toes. As the cells are continually worn away, they are continually replaced by cells from the deeper layers.

The dermis

This is a dense layer of fibrous tissue which is well supplied with blood vessels and nerves.

The skin contains hairs, nails, sweat glands and sebaceous glands.

Hair

One of man's distinctive characteristics is his apparent hairlessness. However, a closer inspection of the skin shows that, even in hairless areas, it is covered with many fine hairs. The only areas completely devoid of hairs are the palms of the hands, soles of the feet, and the lips.

Some hairs have a protective function. The hairs in the nose and ear canal are directed outwards to prevent the entry of foreign objects. The eyelashes guard the eyes in a similar manner.

Nails

The nails have developed as modifications of the skin, to protect the ends of the fingers. All growth of the nail takes place from the root, which is implanted into a groove in the skin. If a nail is injured and removed, without damage to the nail root, a new nail will grow.

Sweat glands

Sweat glands are found in most areas of skin and are situated in the subcutaneous layer. Sweat is carried from the gland along the duct to the surface of the skin where it opens onto the skin through a pore. The sweat glands play a part in temperature control by the evaporation of sweat from the surface of the skin. They not only react to an increase in temperature, but are supplied with autonomic nerve fibres and react to stressful situations by producing sweat.

Sebaceous glands

These open onto each hair follicle and secrete an oily substance called sebum, which acts as a lubricant and possibly a nutrient for the hair shaft. It also serves a protective function on the skin by keeping it soft and supple, and acting as a weak antiseptic.

FUNCTIONS OF THE SKIN

(1) Regulation of body temperature,
(2) Provision of a barrier to infection,
(3) Transmission of sensations from the environment,
(4) Protection of the body from excessive exposure to sunlight

Regulation of body temperature

The skin acts as a thermostat by helping to control the body temperature at about 36.9 °C (98.4 °F). The central control of body temperature is in the brain, but a rise in body temperature produces an increase in blood flow to the skin, increasing heat loss. Sweating is produced – because the heat loss is increased further by water evaporating from the wet skin.

When the temperature falls, blood supply to the skin is reduced and the skin becomes pale and cold.

Provision of a barrier to infection

The scaly nature of the skin surface acts as a deterrent against bacteria and helps to prevent them getting into the tissues. The weak antiseptic secretion, sebum, produced by the sebaceous glands, also protects the skin. The tissues become vulnerable once the skin surface is broken by a wound.

Transmission of sensations from the environment

Skin is well supplied with nerves, which are mostly sensory. They transmit the different sensations of pain, touch, heat and cold. If a sensory nerve is cut, sensation is lost in the area of skin supplied by that nerve. During recovery the area affected gets smaller, until sensation returns.

Touch corpuscles are very numerous in areas specially sensitive to touch – such as the fingertips. They are stimulated by pressure on the skin.

Sensations of 'hot' and 'cold' are felt at certain points on the skin, so called 'hot spots' and 'cold spots'.

The skin is therefore well supplied with a range of analysers to sort out the various sensations received from the environment and to transmit information about them to the brain.

Protection of the body from excessive exposure to sunlight

The colour of skin results mainly from a brown pigment, melanin, in the deeper layers of the epidermis. Melanin protects the body by absorbing radiation in sunlight. Even in white races, the skin contains melanin and the amount of melanin is increased in prolonged exposure to sunlight. Complete absence of melanin occurs in an albino – affecting not only the skin, but the eyes and hair as well.

INFLAMMATION

Inflammation is the response of living tissues to injury, caused by trauma, heat, infection or chemicals. The local effects are shown by heat, redness, pain and swelling.

Once a source of inflammation is present, the body attempts to counter it by calling on its defence mechanisms. The blood vessels dilate, increasing the blood flow to the affected area. This brings large numbers of white cells to the area and they pass through the capillary wall to deal with any bacteria present in the tissues. The surrounding tissues produce a fluid (exudate) which may help in diluting any toxin produced by the bacteria.

The body's inflammatory reaction is a protective reaction and is more effective if the agent is overcome and the reaction remains localized. This is more likely to happen if the area involved is well supplied with blood vessels. The skin can protect itself well – because of its rich blood supply, whereas the cornea has no blood vessels and is very vulnerable to invading bacteria.

The outcome of inflammation is dependent on the balance between the body's ability to defend itself and the power of the bacteria to overcome those defences. The outcome may be complete resolution and recovery – or breakdown of tissue, with the production of pus and abscess formation. If the defence reaction is overwhelmed, the inflammatory process and the invading agent will spread locally and generally to affect the rest of the body. Infection of the bloodstream (septicaemia) may result in death.

3
The respiratory system and asphyxia

RESPIRATION

Respiration is the process which enables oxygen to be absorbed into the bloodstream. At the same time carbon dioxide is removed from the bloodstream and expelled from the body, through the lungs.

The air travels through the nose, pharynx, larynx, trachea and bronchi to reach the lungs, where the gas exchange takes place (Figure 3.1).

In the nose the air is warmed and moistened. Any large particles are trapped by cells lining the nasal cavity. These cells have hairs, called cilia, which move rather like a field of corn waving in the wind and gradually move the large particles out towards the nostrils. Smaller particles which manage to get through the nasal cavity are eventually trapped on similar cells further down the respiratory system. A similar action of the cilia, aided by a sticky mucus and coughing, enables the particles to be brought up to the pharynx and they are then either swallowed or coughed out. The sinuses are in direct communication with the nasal cavity and are used in the production of voice resonance. This action is hampered when the sinuses become infected during episodes of sinusitis.

The pharynx is composed of:

(1) the nasopharynx leading from the nasal cavity,

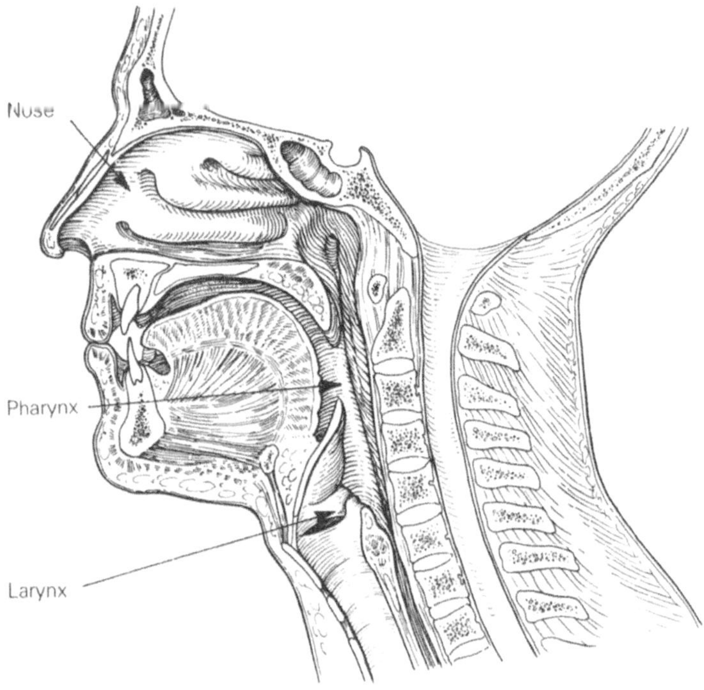

Figure 3.1 The nose, pharynx and larynx

(2) the oropharynx leading from the back of the mouth.

The oropharynx is occupied by the tongue, which is a relatively large muscular organ. Because of its size and position it is easy for the tongue to slip back and block the airway, causing an obstruction in the pharynx. The larynx is situated within the thyroid cartilage, which is also known as Adam's Apple. It contains the vocal cords and it is here that the voice is produced.

The trachea is a tube which leads from the larynx to the bronchi (Figure 3.2). It is strengthened by rings of cartilage which prevent the tube from collapsing. The trachea divides into the right and left bronchi, and each bronchus divides into branches which go to each lobe of the lung. The right lung has three lobes, whereas the left lung has only two lobes – to allow for the space taken up by the heart. The lungs are grey, but become darker during life as a result of inhaled dust and particles of carbon.

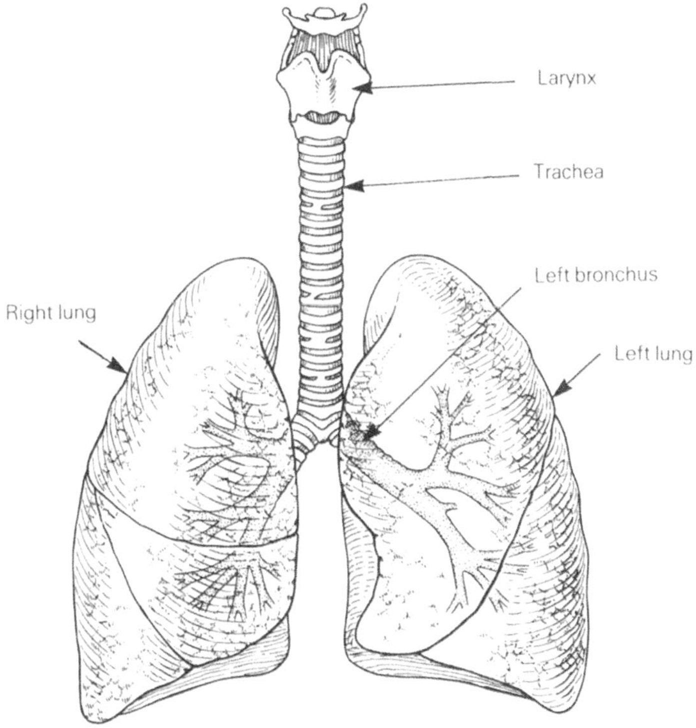

Figure 3.2 The trachea and lungs

The lungs are protected by the rib cage (Figure 3.3). They are covered by a membrane, called the pleura, and this is reflected onto the inside of the chest wall. A small amount of lubricant fluid produced by the two layers of the pleura allows the lungs to move smoothly within the chest wall while they inflate and deflate. Inside the substance of the lungs the bronchi divide into smaller branches, called bronchioles, which themselves become smaller and smaller. The whole structure resembles an inverted tree and is called the bronchial tree. The smallest bronchioles eventually end in air sacs called alveoli, which are thin-walled structures covered

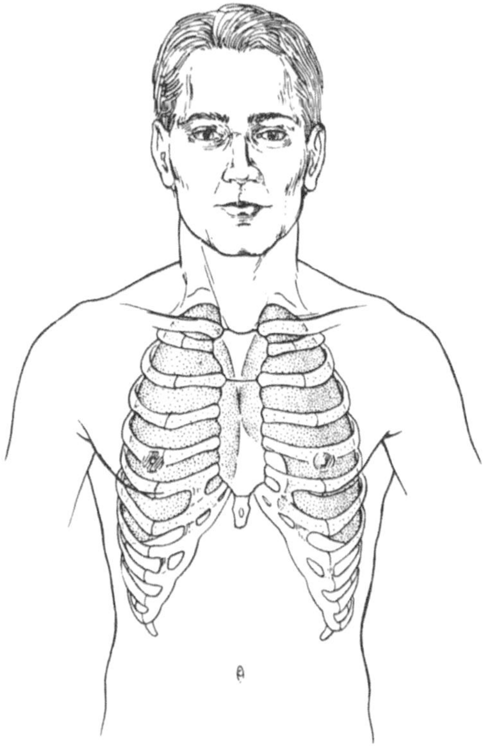

Figure 3.3 The rib cage protecting the lungs

by capillaries from the pulmonary circulation.

The gas exchange of oxygen and carbon dioxide takes place through the walls of the alveoli (Figure 3.4). The deoxygenated blood is brought to the lungs from the heart by the pulmonary artery. The carbon dioxide leaves the bloodstream and passes into the alveoli. Oxygen leaves the alveoli and passes into the bloodstream. The oxygenated blood is returned to the heart by the pulmonary vein.

This situation, the link between the heart and the lungs, is unique in that it is the only situation in the body where an *artery* (the pulmonary artery) (Figure 3.5(a)) carries *deoxygenated* blood and a *vein* (the pulmonary vein) (Figure 3.5(b)) carries *oxygenated* blood.

The mechanism of respiration is produced by the diaphragm and the intercostal muscles. The diaphragm is the main muscle of respiration and is situated at the base of the chest cavity. (Figure 3.6).

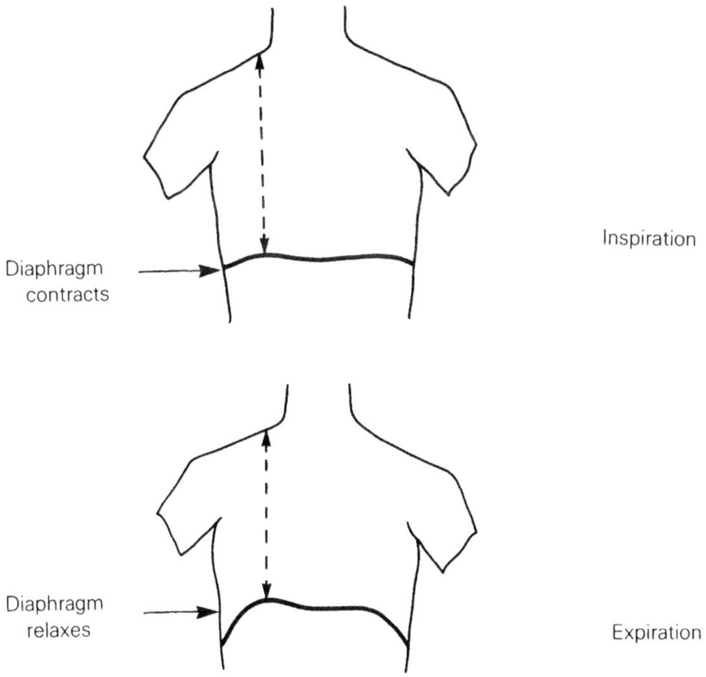

Figure 3.6 The mechanism of respiration produced by the diaphragm

When the diaphragm contracts it increases the volume of the chest cavity and air is drawn into the chest. When the diaphragm relaxes, the volume of the chest cavity is reduced and the natural elasticity of the lungs allows the air to be expelled. The intercostal muscles are situated between the ribs, and when they contract they pull each rib upwards and outwards. This action also increases the size of the chest cavity in inspiration. When the respiratory effort is increased, for example both during and after exertion, additional muscles in the neck attached to the chest wall, and also the abdominal muscles, may be called into action.

The control of breathing can be:

(1) voluntary,
(2) automatic – under the control of the respiratory centre which is situated in the brain stem.

The respiratory centre is stimulated by an increasing level of carbon dioxide in the blood and its activity is reduced by drugs. During, and after, strenuous physical exercise the respiratory rate increases, until the level of carbon dioxide in the blood falls to a normal level.

The breathing rate depends on the body's requirement for oxygen and in a person who is at rest the rate may vary between 12 and 18 breaths per minute.

Tissue respiration

When oxygen reaches the tissues it is given up to the cells, and carbon dioxide is taken by the blood in exchange. This exchange of gases at the tissues takes place at the capillaries, which have very thin walls, to allow gases to pass through easily.

ASPHYXIA

Asphyxia is a condition where there is a lack of oxygen in the blood. The brain requires a constant supply of oxygen to function normally. If a lack of oxygen exists for longer than 4 minutes irreversible brain damage may occur.

Asphyxia may be caused by:

(1) a lack of oxygen in the air,
(2) obstruction of the airway,
(3) chest or lung damage,
(4) conditions affecting the respiratory centre and respiratory muscles,
(5) an inability to use oxygen.

Lack of available oxygen

There may be no oxygen available in the air. It may have been replaced by a poisonous gas such as carbon monoxide (see P.81). Alternatively, oxygen may be present, but it may be at the wrong pressure. Mountaineers require a supplementary supply of oxygen, in the form of oxygen cylinders, when they climb the highest mountains.

Obstruction of the airway

External pressure

External pressure can be applied from strangling, hanging and smothering with a pillow. Polythene bags are a potential cause of asphyxia if a child is allowed to play with them and put one over his head. A warning is usually printed on large polythene bags to prevent a possible catastrophe.

Tongue

This may slip back and block the airway in a casualty who is unconscious, as the unconscious casualty has no control over his own airway. Attention to the position of the jaw, and, if necessary, hooking the tongue forwards should relieve the asphyxia.

Foreign body

This includes food, false teeth and vomit. The foreign body should be removed from the airway as quickly as possible.

Blood from an injury to the airway

Haemorrhage should be controlled as quickly as possible and, if the blood is causing an obstruction to the airway, it should be removed.

Chest or lung damage

External pressure

External pressure on the chest wall can be caused from the casualty being trapped in machinery, or by falling masonry. If the casualty cannot be freed quickly, an attempt should be made to overcome asphyxia by commencing resuscitation immediately by whichever method is appropriate under the circumstances.

Perforating wounds of the chest wall

In this situation air may enter the pleural cavity, resulting in collapse of the lung and a potential 'sucking wound', where air is drawn into the pleural cavity on inspiration, but is not released through the wound on expiration. The longer the sucking wound is allowed to persist, the more air is drawn into the pleural cavity. This increases the casualty's distress and breathing becomes shallow and difficult.

Blast injury

A bomb explosion, or explosion caused by the ignition of a combustible gas, produces many small haemorrhages in the lungs. The lungs are unable to function efficiently and the casualty may become asphyxiated. He may cough up some frothy blood. He must be examined for other injuries – as he may be suffering from burns, fractures or perforated ear-drums. Immediate transport to hospital is required.

Drowning

Obviously the lungs will not function satisfactorily when they are full of water. Artificial respiration should be commenced as soon as possible – if necessary whilst the casualty is still in deep water. Further inhalations should be given when both casualty and rescuer have reached a position of support in the water. When the casualty is out of the water resuscitation should be continued while transport to hospital is being arranged.

Conditions affecting the respiratory centre and muscles

Tetanus

This is a disease caused by tetanus spores gaining entry to the body through a dirty wound. The spores produce a toxin which affects the muscles of the body, causing spasm. When those muscles are the muscles of respiration, the casualty becomes asphyxiated and requires treatment with a respirator.

Poisons and drugs

These have a depressant effect on the respiratory centre in the brain and slow down the rate of respiration.

Electrocution

Electricity passing through the body may cause respiration to stop suddenly, in association with the heart stopping. Care should be taken to ensure that the electricity is switched off or the casualty removed from the source of the electricity, using a non-conducting material, before any attempt at resuscitation is made.

Head and spinal injury

If the spinal cord is damaged in the neck, the nerves supplying the diaphragm and the intercostal muscles may be affected, producing muscular paralysis.

Inability to use oxygen

Even if the respiratory system is working adequately and oxygen is available for use by the body, it may be unable to use the oxygen, as in:

(1) Coronary thrombosis, where the heart muscle is damaged to such an extent that there is 'pump failure', and the blood is not pumped around the body to enable the oxygen to be delivered to the tissues.

(2) Cyanide poisoning, where cyanide prevents the tissues from taking up the oxygen supplied to them by the bloodstream.

The symptoms of asphyxia are:

(1) jerky, irregular breathing,
(2) coughing,
(3) cyanosis – the fingertips, ear-lobes and lips become blue,
(4) the casualty may become unconscious.

The asphyxiating casualty may not necessarily have stopped breathing. Any obvious cause of asphyxia should be removed, or the casualty removed from the cause. If, despite this, the casualty's breathing it still distressed, it is possible to give 'assisted' breathing while waiting for the emergency services.

EXTRICATION FROM GAS OR CHEMICAL FILLED AREAS

A casualty who is trapped in a gas or chemical filled area will rapidly become asphyxiated. Unless he is removed from that area and artificial respiration commenced within 4 minutes, irreversible brain damage may occur.

The first-aider must assess the situation and not rush immediately to the aid of the victim – risking the same fate as the victim. If specially-trained personnel are readily available they should obviously be used to rescue the casualty.

However, it should be remembered that speed is of great importance and the casualty must be removed from the area as quickly as possible. If the situation is the result of an industrial accident there may be protective clothing and a gas mask or breathing apparatus for the rescuer to wear. If this is not available the rescuer should put a handkerchief over the mouth and nose, and approach the casualty along the floor in the hope that the gas or chemical involved will be lighter than air and will therefore accumulate in the upper part of the room.

In all cases the rescuer should be linked by rope to another person, as a safety procedure in case he gets into difficulties.

A casualty who is recovering from asphyxia is very likely to vomit and he should therefore be placed in the recovery position during transit to hospital. The airway should be continually monitored.

CHOKING

Choking occurs when a foreign body inadvertently enters the respiratory system. Partial choking is a fairly common event and occurs when 'food goes down the wrong way'. The casualty has a spasm of coughing and develops a livid or cyanosed appearance. If unrelieved the condition quickly leads to unconsciousness and death. The object is to remove the foreign body before irreversible brain damage occurs. If it is in the pharynx and is large and accessible, it should be removed quickly. If the foreign body has reached further down the respiratory system, the treatment is as follows:

Infant	—	Hold up by the legs and smack between the shoulders.
Child	—	Lay across the knee and slap between the shoulders.
Adult	—	Three or four blows between the shoulders with the head lowered.

This method of removing the foreign body is the one to be used first. Unfortunately the foreign body will some-times be dislodged rather than expelled, and may impact against the vocal cords – increasing the problem. An alternative method removes the foreign body by means of an abdominal thrust, and is known as the Heimlich manoeuvre.

The Heimlich manoeuvre (or abdominal thrust)

The Heimlich manoeuvre was first described in 1974 by Professor Henry Heimlich in America. He became aware of choking as a major cause of accidental death and realized that foreign body obstruction of the airway usually occurs while the victim is eating. He undertook research to devise a method which would effectively remove the airway obstruction. Speed is essential as the obstruction must be removed within 4 minutes.

The initial task for the rescuer is to recognize the situation in terms of potential choking. A child who is running while eating, or an infant who is allowed to play with small toys or beads – both have the ingredients for a choking incident. Many cases of choking in restaurants have been successfully relieved by the Heimlich manoeuvre.

The second task for the rescuer is to recognize the choking victim (Figure 3.7). The victim may bring the hand to the throat, giving the Heimlich sign to indicate choking. The thumb and index finger form a V at the neck. The sign tends to be given instinctively. The casualty cannot speak and may give jerky attempts to breathe. He becomes cyanosed and may become unconscious.

If the choking incident occurs in the setting of a formal dinner

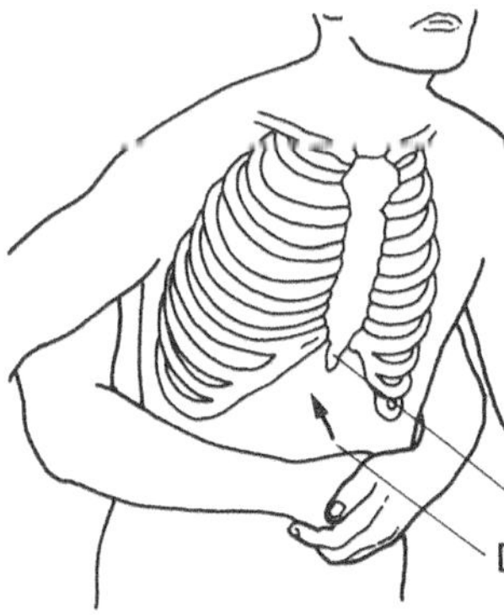

Figure 3.7 The Heimlich manoeuvre – position of the rescuer's hands

party, or a crowded restaurant, the victim may become very embarrassed by his predicament and attempt to leave the table and go to the toilet. If the choking is not relieved, he rapidly becomes cyanosed and unconscious in an area where he may unfortunately be alone – with fatal consequences.

The reason the Heimlich manoeuvre is so successful is that no matter what phase of respiration the victim is in when choking occurs, there is still a considerable volume of air remaining in the lungs. When the abdominal thrust is applied below the diaphragm, air is expelled and this forces the obstructing object out of the airway (Figure 3.8).

The technique of the Heimlich manoeuvre

The Heimlich manoeuvre can be used when the victim is standing, sitting or lying on the floor. When the victim is standing, the rescuer stands behind him and puts his arms around the victim's waist (Figure 3.9). With one hand he makes a fist and places the thumb against the victim's abdomen, below the sternum and above the umbilicus. With a quick upward thrust the rescuer presses into the victim's abdomen. It may be necessary to repeat the manoeuvre several times to clear the airway. If the foreign body has been removed adequately the casualty will resume normal breathing and there will be a return to normal colour.

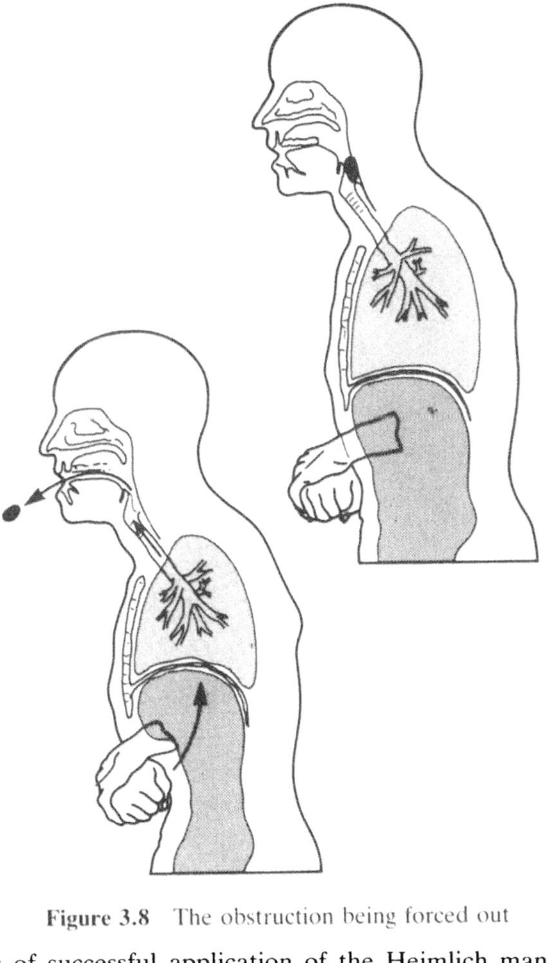

Figure 3.8 The obstruction being forced out

Reports of successful application of the Heimlich manoeuvre indicate that the foreign body is expelled from the airway with some force, but if this does not happen, a search for the foreign body should be made in the pharynx and it should be manually removed. Great care should be taken that the attempt at removal does not force the foreign body back into the airway.

If the victim is seated when the Heimlich manoeuvre is performed, the rescuer positions his hands in exactly the same way. The back of the chair provides a firm support for the victim's back and there may be some enhanced thrust by using the back of

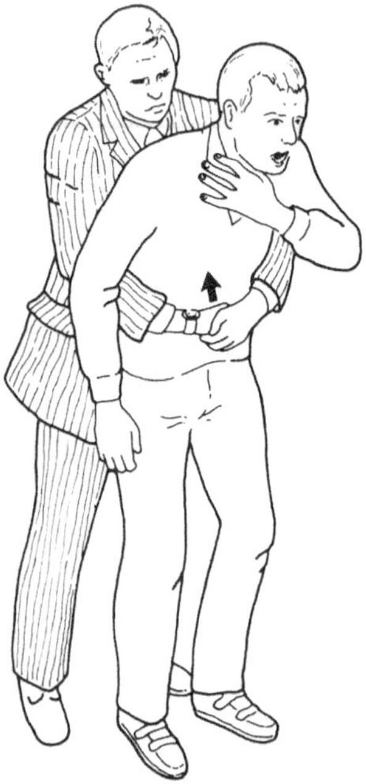

Figure 3.9 The Heimlich manoeuvre on a standing casualty

the chair as a support.

If the casualty is unconscious, or the first-aider is small or weak, the Heimlich manoeuvre can be performed with the victim lying on the floor. The principle is exactly the same, but the first-aider kneels astride the victim and places the hands one on top of the other, just below the sternum and above the umbilicus. The direction of force is again towards the diaphragm.

It is possible for the Heimlich manoeuvre to be self-administered. The victim can use his own hands in the correct position to administer the thrust, or he could use the back of a chair to provide the force.

In the case of an infant the victim is held on the rescuer's lap and the force is produced by directing the index and middle fingers of both hands below the sternum towards the diaphragm.

It is hoped that the wider application of the Heimlich manoeuvre will result in fewer deaths from choking.

ASTHMA

Asthma is a condition where there is reversible airways obstruction – improving spontaneously or in response to drug treatment.

Asthma can start at any age, but the incidence is highest in children and middle age. There is *usually* an hereditary link in the production of asthma. There is *often* an allergic basis for the symptoms and there is *occasionally* a psychological factor which aggravates the condition.

Various factors may be responsible for initiating an episode of asthma:

(1) viral and bacterial respiratory infections,
(2) dust, pollen,
(3) drugs and food (eggs, milk, fish),
(4) exercise
(5) stress – including anger and excitement.

Asthma is characterized by episodes of shortness of breath accompanied by wheezing. This is produced by a temporary narrowing of the bronchi by muscle spasm and an accumulation of bronchial secretions. The efficiency of the lungs is reduced and the patient may become very distressed in his effort to get sufficient air into the lungs.

A typical episode of asthma, which may occur at any time of the day or night, occurs rather suddenly and may be preceded by a tight feeling in the chest. Breathing out becomes difficult and wheezing is heard. In contrast to the difficulty in expiration, inspiration is short and gasping. The patient remains in a sitting position, in an attempt to fix the shoulder girdle and assist the accessory muscles of respiration. There is an increasing difficulty in talking because of respiratory distress. There is often an unproductive cough which aggravates the shortness of breath. The pulse becomes rapid and cyanosis may develop.

First aid management of asthma

About 1000 people die from acute asthma in England and Wales each year, either suddenly in an acute attack, or after slowly developing increasingly severe asthma – which was underestimated by people around them.

The casualty will be in a distressed condition and will require reassurance. He should be placed in a sitting position, which will help the lungs to work as efficiently as the difficult circumstances will allow.

If he is a known asthmatic he may have some treatment readily available in the form of an inhaler. He should be encouraged to use this to overcome the wheezing. If there is no early sign of improvement, medical help should be obtained as quickly as possible.

It is much easier to relieve an episode of asthma in the early stages of wheezing, rather than delay treatment and attempt to relieve the symptoms when the wheezing has been present for many hours.

ANGINA AND CORONARY THROMBOSIS

The first branches from the aorta are the coronary arteries supplying blood to the muscle of the heart. Being a muscular organ the heart relies on the blood flow along the coronary arteries to supply it with oxygen and nourishment for its continued activity. Throughout life the coronary arteries may become narrowed and this reduces the blood flow – producing coronary artery disease.

One of the striking features of life in the western world this century is the high incidence of coronary artery disease. It is one of the most common causes of death. Several factors play a part in the incidence of coronary artery disease – high intake of animal fat, cigarette smoking, lack of exercise and obesity.

Narrowing of the coronary arteries may increase to such an extent that the blood flow is severely restricted. During exercise the blood flow may not be sufficient for the oxygen requirement of the heart muscle, and the characteristic chest pain of angina is produced. If a clot, or thrombus, develops in the coronary artery the blood supply to part of the heart muscle is cut off.

Angina

Pain characteristic of angina is precipitated by exercise or emotion – especially after a heavy meal or in cold weather. The casualty complains of a tight, cramp-like or vice-like pain behind the sternum, and moving upwards to the throat, jaw and one or both arms. If he is exercising, running or walking the pain makes him stop. It is relieved within a few minutes by resting. If he suffers from frequent episodes of angina he may be accustomed to relieving the pain by placing an anti-angina tablet under the tongue.

Most patients, by adjusting the way they live and by using drugs, manage to cope satisfactorily with the limitations imposed by angina. Occasionally the symptoms become incapacitating and a coronary artery bypass graft operation may be performed, using a vein from the patient's leg to bypass the narrowed section of the coronary artery.

Coronary thrombosis

For a person who has narrowed coronary arteries there is always the risk that a clot may form in the narrowed blood vessel and suddenly stop the blood supply to a section of heart muscle.

A coronary thrombosis may occur at any time, day or night, during exercise or even at rest. It begins with sudden, severe chest pain of the same type and distribution as angina, and usually lasting for several hours.

The casualty may collapse, having had a cardiac arrest. Resuscitation is required and medical help sought. If death does not occur at the outset, the casualty is at greatest risk of death in the first 2 hours.

Complications of coronary thrombosis

Heart failure This occurs when the efficiency of the heart is affected by damage to the heart muscle. It produces shortness of breath and cyanosis. The casualty should be placed in a sitting position and urgent transport to hospital arranged.

Shock Extensive damage to the heart muscle produces the signs and symptoms of shock. Raising the foot of the bed is often regarded as beneficial – but may be contraindicated in the presence of heart failure.

Irregular heart action This is the main factor in a large percentage of the deaths in the few hours immediately after the coronary thrombosis. For this reason a casualty suffering from a coronary thrombosis should receive urgent medical attention, perhaps including emergency admission to hospital.

THEORY OF RESUSCITATION

The object of resuscitation is to restore an oxygenated blood supply to the brain and major organs of the body. This must be achieved within 4 minutes, otherwise irreversible brain damage will occur.

The three components of emergency resuscitation are:

(1) *The airway,* which must be kept patent to allow air to reach the lungs for gas exchange,

(2) *Breathing,* which must be adequate to allow sufficient oxygen to be drawn into the lungs,

(3) *Circulation,* which must be capable of carrying oxygenated blood to all parts of the body.

Artificial respiration

Where artificial respiration is required, the mouth-to-mouth method is the method of choice. This method is convenient and easy to perform. It uses the expired air of the first-aider to provide oxygen for the casualty and delivers the oxygen directly into the casualty's airway. The efficiency of the method can be monitored by observing the casualty's chest wall rise and fall during the application of the method. The reason it is so successful can be seen from the constituents of fresh air and expired air (Table 3.1).

Table 3.1 Constituents of fresh and expired air

Fresh air	%	*Expired air*	%
Nitrogen	79.00	Nitrogen	79.0
Oxygen	20.96	Oxygen	16.5
Carbon dioxide	0.04	Carbon dioxide	4.5

While the quantity of nitrogen remains the same in both fresh air and expired air, the amount of carbon dioxide increases ten-fold in the expired air, whereas the amount of oxygen falls from 20.96% to 16.5% in the expired air. For a victim who is asphyxiated, and therefore suffering from lack of oxygen, 16.5% oxygen is very useful to receive and can indeed be life saving.

External cardiac compression

External cardiac compression must be started only when there is no carotid pulse detectable at the neck. The pupils may begin to dilate.

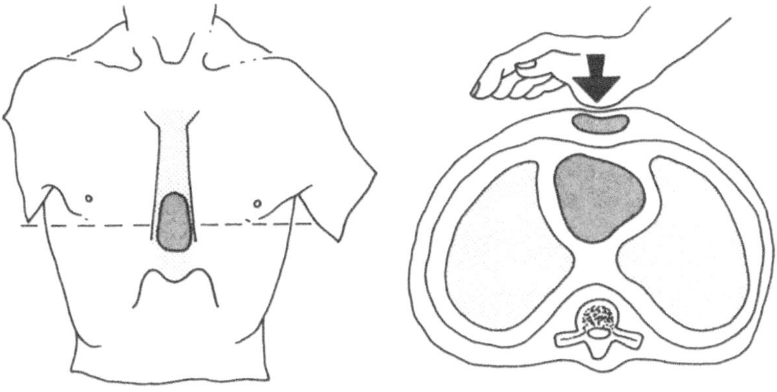

Figure 3.10 External cardiac compression

The object of external cardiac compression is to empty the blood from the heart by squeezing it between the sternum and the vertebral column (Figure 3.10). To achieve this the casualty should be on his back on a hard surface – and not on a soft mattress. The force of the compression should be strong enough to produce a pulse in the carotid artery. The rate of the compression should be 60–80 per minute and with artificial respiration should effectively be 5 to 1 or 15 to 2 depending on the number of first-aiders involved.

Resuscitation should continue while there is any hope that the heart will beat spontaneously again. Help should be requested and, if necessary, resuscitation should continue until the casualty arrives at hospital.

4
The circulation, haemorrhage and shock

BLOOD AND THE CIRCULATION

Blood is the fluid contained in the circulatory system. There are approximately 6 litres (10 pints) of blood in the adult male body although this varies according to size of the casualty. It also depends on the age of the casualty and a young child may only have one or two pints of blood. Blood is composed of red cells, white cells and platelets floating in fluid called plasma (Figure 4.1).

The *red cells*, of which there are five million per cubic millimetre of blood, contain a pigment called haemoglobin. This is used as the transport system for oxygen in the body and combines with oxygen in the red cells. Unfortunately this transport system is disrupted in a case of carbon monoxide poisoning. Haemoglobin has a much greater affinity for carbon monoxide which will bind to haemoglobin forming carboxyhaemoglobin at the expense of oxygen. The patient will therefore become asphyxiated. If the number of red cells falls either by repeated blood loss or a failure of red cell production in the bone marrow, anaemia may develop.

The *white cells*, or leukocytes, defend the body against attack by infection. They number about 6–10 thousand per cubic millimetre of blood. When infection is present the number of white cells will increase. The combination of bacteria, debris and white cells produces pus at the site of infection. The *platelets* are much smaller than the other cells and are concerned with the process of blood clotting. Apart from these functions blood also carries nutrient materials and waste products, such as carbon dioxide, from the tissues to various organs, and it circulates heat in order to maintain a fairly constant body temperature.

The blood circulates in the blood vessels, with the arteries carrying the blood away from the heart to the tissues, and the veins returning it to the heart (Figure 4.2). The major arteries, which are thick-walled structures, divide into smaller and smaller arteries. The smallest arteries, called arterioles, eventually divide into very thin-walled structures called capillaries. These are thin enough to allow oxygen, carbon dioxide and nutrients to pass from the blood to the tissues, and vice versa. Several capillaries then merge to form small veins, called venules, and these form larger and larger veins, carrying the blood, eventually, to the heart. Veins are thin-walled structures, and, unlike arteries, contain valves at various points *en route* to the heart. These prevent any reverse flow of blood and so maintain a one-way flow through the circulatory system.

THE HEART

The heart is a muscular organ which acts as a pump for the circulation. The pumping action is built into the muscle of the heart and can be modified by the involuntary nerve control to the heart muscle. In the major arteries, such as the carotid artery in the neck and the radial artery in the wrists, the pumping action can be registered as the pulse. In a normal healthy adult the pulse rate is 60–80 beats per minute. Exercise, illness and shock will increase the pulse rate. It is also faster in babies (100–120 beats per minute).

The pulse rate will be slower in people who do a lot of regular physical training. In this group it can be 50–60 beats per minute.

The pulse is normally regular but may become irregular with illness or anything which produces an inefficient heart action. The irregular pulse may have been present for many years in an otherwise healthy individual – and in that case may be a relic of a past illness.

The heart is situated in the centre and left side of the chest (Figure 4.3). It is about the size of an adult male clenched fist. The apex of the heart can be felt on the chest wall just below the left nipple.

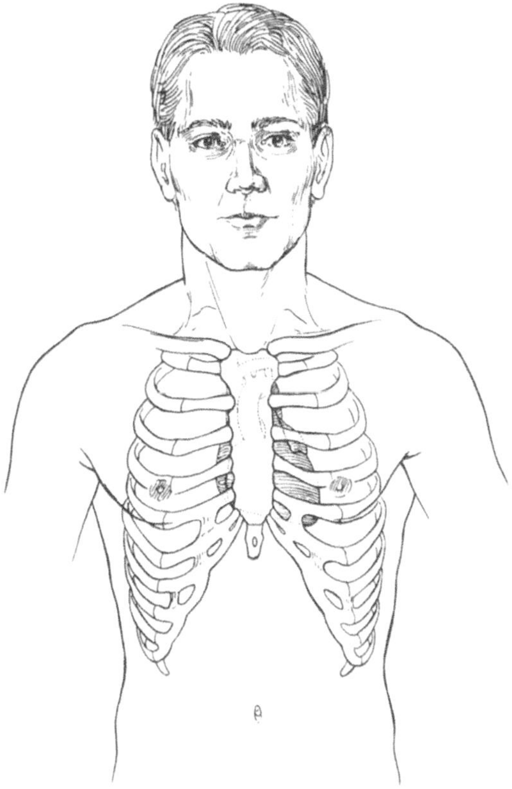

Figure 4.3 Position of the heart in the chest

The heart is divided into two halves by the septum and each side is divided into two chambers by a valve (Figure 4.4). The upper chamber is the atrium and the lower chamber is the ventricle. The right atrium receives blood returned to the heart by the major veins. The blood passes through the valve into the right ventricle and is pumped towards the lungs by the right ventricle, along the pulmonary arteries. At this point the blood is deoxygenated and this is the only situation in the body where an artery carries deoxygenated blood. In the lungs the blood receives oxygen and gives up carbon dioxide in the process of respiration. The oxygenated blood returns via the pulmonary veins to the left atrium and conversely this is a situation where veins are carrying oxygenated blood. The blood travels through the valve into the left ventricle and is then pumped out of the heart along the aorta, to travel to all parts of the body. This part of the circulation is called the systemic circulation, and that part of the circuit which takes blood to the lungs and back to the heart is the pulmonary circulation.

HAEMORRHAGE

Haemorrhage is usually associated with injury and may be:

(1) external
(2) internal
    (a) revealed – by making its way to the outside,
    (b) concealed – by remaining in a body cavity.

Haemorrhage resulting in concealed internal bleeding means that the blood is still lost to the body, as it is not available for the circulation if it remains in a body cavity, or in the thigh, following a fractured femur.

Haemorrhage may also be arterial, venous or capillary.

Arterial haemorrhage

Bleeding from an artery is bright red and pulsatile – spurting in rhythm with the heart beat. Arterial blood is at a higher pressure than anywhere else in the circulation and this results in more blood being lost.

Arterial bleeding may be:

(1) primary – occurring at the time of injury, or
(2) secondary – occurring about 10 days after injury and usually caused by infection at the site of healing.

Venous haemorrhage

Bleeding from a vein is dark red and occurs in a steady trickle from the blood vessel. The pressure in the vessel is less than in an artery and bleeding can be controlled by reducing the venous pressure even more by elevating the limb and applying direct pressure.

Capillary haemorrhage

This occurs from the smallest blood vessels and produces a gentle oozing from the wound surface.

Effects of haemorrhage

Once haemorrhage has occurred, the body's immediate reaction is to attempt to stop the continuing loss of blood, and to minimize the effects of the haemorrhage on the rest of the body.

Several things happen at the site of bleeding – the ends of the blood vessels contract and narrow, and a clot is produced by the platelets, to act as a plug at the opening in the blood vessel.

The reduction in blood volume reduces the venous return to the heart. The circulation responds by increasing the heart rate in an attempt to maintain the flow of blood at a normal rate.

The haemorrhage produces a general effect on the body resulting in a constriction of the blood vessels supplying the skin, muscles, gut and kidneys – thus maintaining a preferential blood supply to the major organs (brain, heart and lungs). The reduction in blood supply to the skin produces the characteristic pale, cold appearance. Respiration becomes rapid – to increase the flow of venous blood back to the heart. Fluid moves into the capillaries from the tissues to help maintain the circulating blood volume. At the same time, an intense thirst develops to increase the body fluids again, and compensate for the loss. The circulating blood volume is usually restored to normal 24–72 hours after a moderate haemorrhage.

If haemorrhage continues, the circulating blood volume may be reduced to such a low level that it is not sufficient to allow the major organs to function adequately – resulting in unconsciousness and death.

Conditions causing excessive bleeding

(1) Platelet deficiency,
(2) Haemophilia.

Platelet deficiency

Platelets are formed in the bone marrow and have a role in the control of haemorrhage by clumping together to form a platelet plug at the site of injury in a blood vessel. When the number of platelets is low, haemorrhage is likely – but varies between mild bruising or a tiny haemorrhagic rash in the skin, to a severe spontaneous haemorrhage from the mouth or nose, or into the stomach, bowel or brain. Cerebral haemorrhage is the commonest cause of death in platelet deficiency.

Haemophilia

Haemophilia was first described in 1803. It is an inherited bleeding disorder of males which is transmitted by healthy females. It is caused by a deficiency of one of two clotting factors (Factor VIII or Factor IX).

Although the deficiency remains virtually the same, the tendency to bleed fluctuates, and can vary from bleeding into the tissues following very minor injury, or even bleeding spontaneously, to managing to sustain quite severe injury without ill effect.

The characteristic feature of haemophilia is wound bleeding, which may persist for several days. Bleeding from the mouth and nose is common in children, and bleeding from the tooth socket following extraction is also common. There may be a spontaneous haemorrhage into a joint, but this usually happens after a mild injury to the joint.

Local treatment must be given in an attempt to control the haemorrhage, but urgent hospitalization is required – for transfusion with fresh blood or plasma, to replace the deficient clotting factor.

Treatment of external haemorrhage

The effective treatment of external haemorrhage is:

(1) direct pressure at the point of bleeding,
(2) elevation of the limb.

A combination of these two actions should control most cases of external haemorrhage.

Some modification may be required in certain circumstances. Direct pressure can only be applied where there is no foreign body in the wound, and no damage has occurred to major structures beneath the wound. In this situation, pressure should be applied *around* the wound.

Elevation of the limb must not be attempted if the limb is fractured.

Pressure points

If there is severe arterial haemorrhage from a wound on a limb, it may be possible to control the haemorrhage by pressure on the artery supplying the area of the wound, at a point where the artery is in close proximity to bone. There are two pressure points on each side of the body. One point is where the brachial artery runs near the inner aspect of the humerus, and the other pressure point is at the centre of the groin, where the femoral artery can be compressed against the lower part of the pelvis.

Revealed internal haemorrhage

Haemorrhage can occur from any of the body orifices and the amount of blood lost may appear quite alarming. Bleeding from the mouth and nose may be controllable by direct pressure, but bleeding from other sources will require medical attention.

Concealed internal haemorrhage

Concealed internal haemorrhage can produce an emergency life-threatening situation, where the casualty is bleeding severely – but no bleeding is visible. It usually occurs in the abdomen and is often the result of a crushing accident, producing damage to a major organ, such as the liver, spleen or kidney. The casualty complains of pain in the abdomen and fails to show the anticipated recovery following the accident. The symptoms and signs of shock persist and intensify. The pulse becomes very rapid and the casualty becomes extremely restless.

The circumstances of the accident should alert the first-aider to the possibility of concealed internal haemorrhage. It is a very serious condition and requires immediate treatment. Urgent transport to hospital should be arranged, with the casualty on a stretcher. The casualty must not be given anything by mouth, because he may undergo an operation on arrival at hospital.

SHOCK

The term 'shock' is usually applied to a situation where the blood flow to the tissues is inadequate. This reduced blood flow can be caused by:

(1) reduced circulating blood volume,
(2) reduced pumping action of the heart (cardiac output),
(3) increased capacity of the circulation – with a normal blood volume and cardiac output.

There are several causes of circulatory failure – loss of circulating fluid from haemorrhage or burns, and the failure of the muscular action of the heart in coronary thrombosis. Other causes of non-cardiac origin, such as infection, can produce similar signs and symptoms – and therefore any comment about shock should refer to the cause of the shock in order to emphasize the likely management.

Forms of shock

(1) Hypovolaemic,
(2) Cardiogenic,
(3) Neurogenic or low resistance,
(4) Anaphylactic.

Hypovolaemic shock

Hypovolaemia means a reduced circulating blood volume from a loss of body fluids, as in haemorrhage, burns and prolonged diarrhoea and vomiting. Haemorrhage following trauma is the most likely cause of hypovolaemia to be encountered in first aid, but it may also occur in an unrecognized, pre-existing condition, such as a peptic ulcer.

The effect of reducing the volume of circulating blood is to reduce the amount of blood returning to the heart. This reduces the output of blood from the heart (the cardiac output) – and the heart increases its pumping rate in an attempt to maintain the circulation. The pulse rate therefore increases.

To help overcome the difficulty, the vessels in the skin and muscles constrict to allow the major organs (the brain, heart and lungs) to receive a preferential supply of blood to maintain life. This gives the casualty the characteristic appearance in shock, of pallor of the skin and being cold to the touch – because the normal flow of blood to the skin brings warmth to the tissues.

The degree of shock produced depends on the amount of circulating fluid lost by haemorrhage (Table 4.1).

Table 4.1 Degree of shock caused by haemorrhage

	Haemorrhage		
	1 pint	*2–3 pints*	*Over 4 pints*
Colour	Normal	Pale	Deathly pale
Skin	Normal	Cold	Cold and clammy
Pulse	Normal	Increased	Very fast and thready
Breathing	Normal	Increased	Increased and sighing

Other symptoms may be present, namely intense thirst (the body's way of attempting to increase the body fluids), restlessness and, eventually, a loss of consciousness may occur.

The important aspect is that once shock has occurred from severe blood loss, the treatment is to replace the lost blood as soon as possible by transfusion. There must be no delay in getting the casualty to hospital.

Other causes of hyopovolaemia – loss of plasma from burns and loss of body fluids from diarrhoea and vomiting – produce shock over a longer period. In the initial stages the signs and symptoms of shock may be absent. With burn injuries, the likelihood of shock developing can be estimated by assessing the area of body surface involved in the burn wound. Shock is likely to develop if the burn area is more than 15% in an adult or more than 10% in a child. Immediate transport to hospital is required for plasma replacement.

Cardiogenic shock

In cardiogenic shock the heart suddenly becomes an ineffective pump for the circulation. The usual cause is damage to the heart muscle from interference with its own blood supply – as a result of a coronary thrombosis. The blood volume remains the same, but the blood flow to the tissue is inadequate.

In this situation, increasing the body fluids by transfusion or giving drinks is not required – and may be harmful by increasing the blood volume and therefore increasing the work the heart has to do as the circulation pump.

The heart will have difficulty in putting out all the blood returned to it by the venous system, and congestion of the lungs and major organs will develop. The symptoms encountered will be those of shock together with noisy, faster, breathing.

Neurogenic shock or low resistance

In neurogenic shock the blood volume and cardiac output remain the same, but there is a loss of muscle tone in the blood vessels. This increases the diameter, and therefore the capacity, of the blood vessels.

In fainting, caused by intense emotion, the blood vessels become very dilated. Blood pools in the vessels and the blood flow falls. Fortunately fainting results in the person falling to the horizontal position and normal cardiac output is restored.

Another cause is associated with bacterial infection and is due to the effects of an endotoxin produced by the bacteria.

Brain damage may also cause neurogenic shock.

These causes of shock are associated with an increased capacity of the blood vessels, producing a 'low resistance' to the blood flow. This is sometimes known as 'warm shock' as there is no constriction of the blood vessels to produce the pale, cold appearance of the skin usually associated with shock. The casualty has a warm flushed skin and develops a rise in temperature, with a bounding pulse.

Anaphylactic shock

Anaphylactic shock is a severe reaction which occurs when a person who has previously been sensitized by a substance (antigen) is exposed to the same substance again.

It can appear within a few minutes of an injection or insect sting. The patient complains of a feeling of uneasiness and becomes restless and hot. Other symptoms may include:

(1) generalized rash,
(2) swelling around the eyes,
(3) red eyes,
(4) wheezy breathing,
(5) increased pulse rate,
(6) vomiting.

Treatment of shock

The treatment of shock should ensure that the cause is corrected and that the body is given some help in its attempt to compensate for the difficulty. When the casualty becomes shocked through haemorrhage, the immediate reaction by the body is to divert blood away from the tissues which do not have an immediate need for a full blood supply, so that the vital organs (brain, lungs and heart) can be supplied. The blood supply to the skin and muscles becomes severely restricted.

The casualty should be quickly examined, and if haemorrhage is present this should be controlled. The airway, respiration and pulse should be checked, and resuscitation given if necessary.

Place the casualty on the floor and elevate the legs if there is no evidence of fracture of the legs. This will increase the venous return to the heart and promote an increased cerebral blood flow. The head should be turned to one side to protect the airway in case the casualty should vomit. If the casualty is repeatedly vomiting, he should be placed in the recovery position.

Prevent the casualty getting cold. If he is shivering, or complaining of being cold, he should be covered with a blanket. Care should be taken not to overheat the casualty as this will dilate the blood vessels in the skin and defeat the object of promoting blood flow to the major organs, by simply diverting blood back again to the skin and muscles.

The casualty may complain of thirst, but drinks should not be given. They may produce vomiting and will delay the administration of an anaesthetic in hospital if further medical treatment is required.

Respiration, pulse rate, level of consciousness and the control of haemorrhage should be checked at frequent intervals. Urgent transport to hospital should be arranged.

5
The nervous system

The nervous system is the communication network which links all parts of the body.

It consists of:

(1) the *central nervous system* which controls voluntary movement and sensation in the body tissues, as well as the special senses and higher mental powers,

(2) the *autonomic nervous system* which controls involuntary movements and activity in the internal organs.

THE CENTRAL NERVOUS SYSTEM

The central nervous system consists of the brain, spinal cord and nerves (Figure 5.1). It is composed of white and grey matter. The white matter consists of nerve fibres and the grey matter consists of nerve cells.

The brain lies within the skull and is the main control unit for the central nervous system. It receives all messages and sensations, gives instructions to the voluntary muscles, registers the special senses and is the centre for consciousness, intelligence and memory. It is comparatively large – its large size distinguishes man from other animals. The surface of the brain is convoluted to increase its surface area. Every part of the body is registered as one point on the surface of the brain.

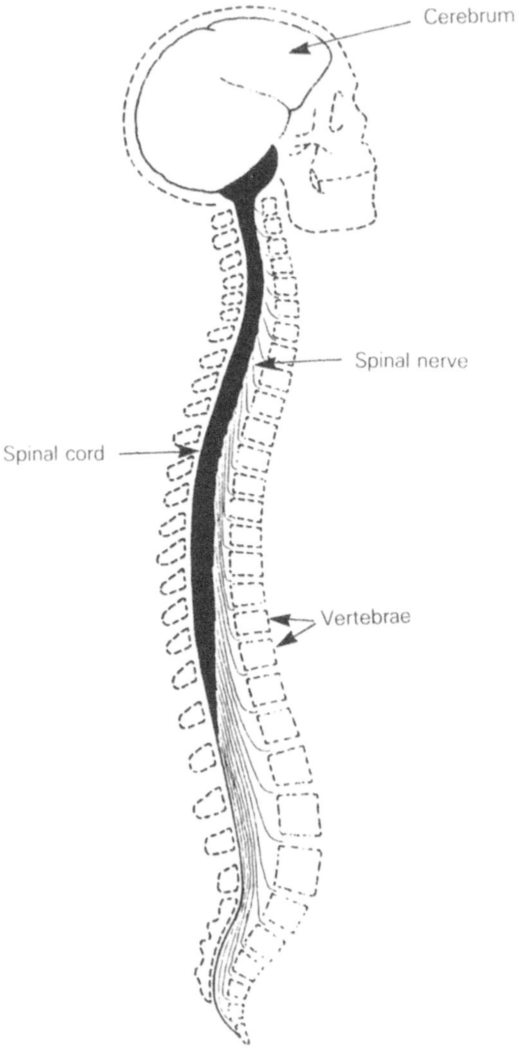

Figure 5.1 The central nervous system

The brain is covered by membranes called meninges. Between the meninges is the cerebrospinal fluid, which provides a cushion effect of protection to the brain.

Twelve pairs of cranial nerves arise from the brain and pass through openings in the skull. They all have a specialized function

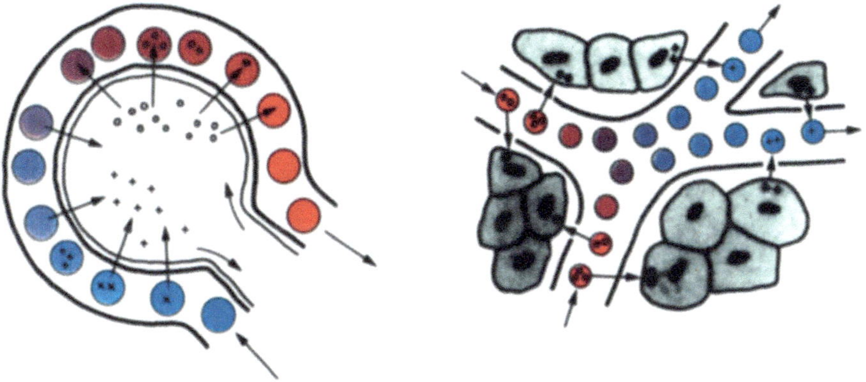

Figure 3.4 The gas exchange of oxygen and carbon dioxide in the alveoli and tissue

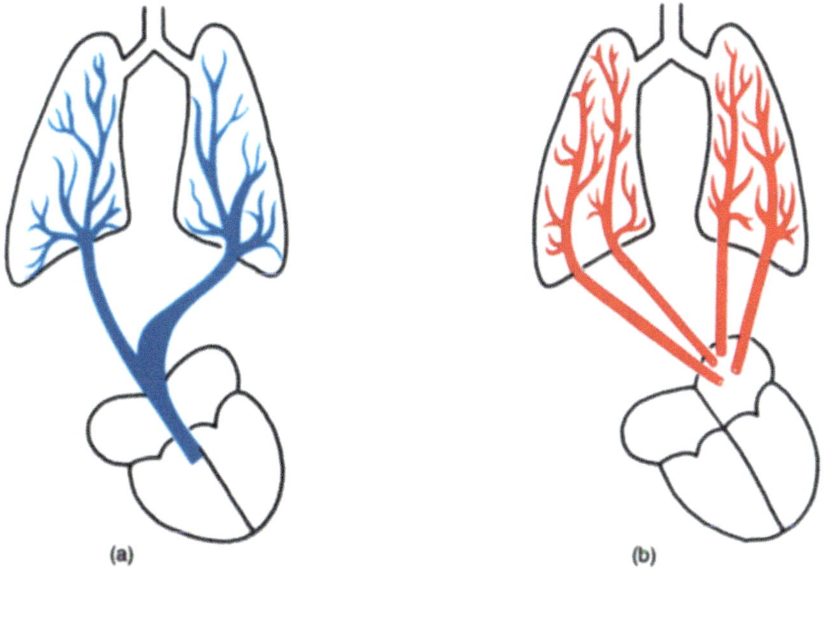

Figure 3.5(a) The pulmonary artery carrying deoxygenated blood; (b) the pulmonary veins carrying oxygenated blood

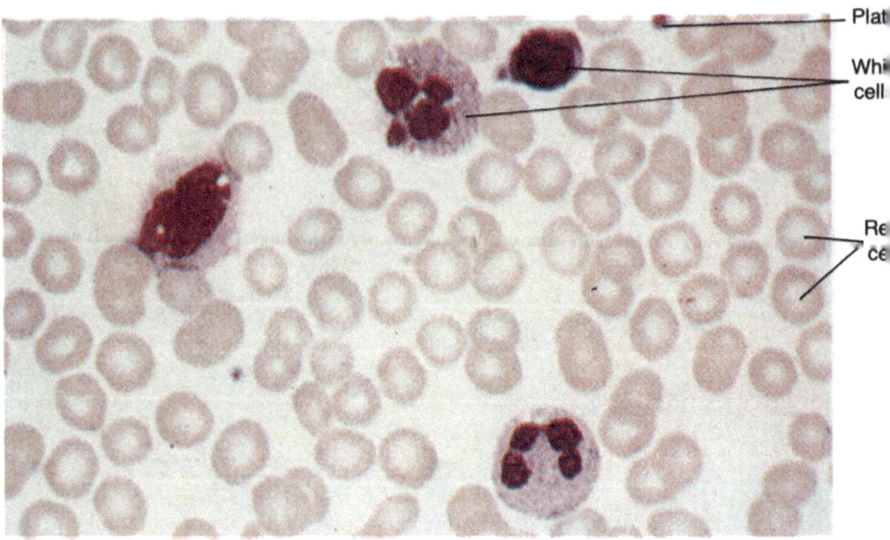

Figure 4.1 Composition of blood

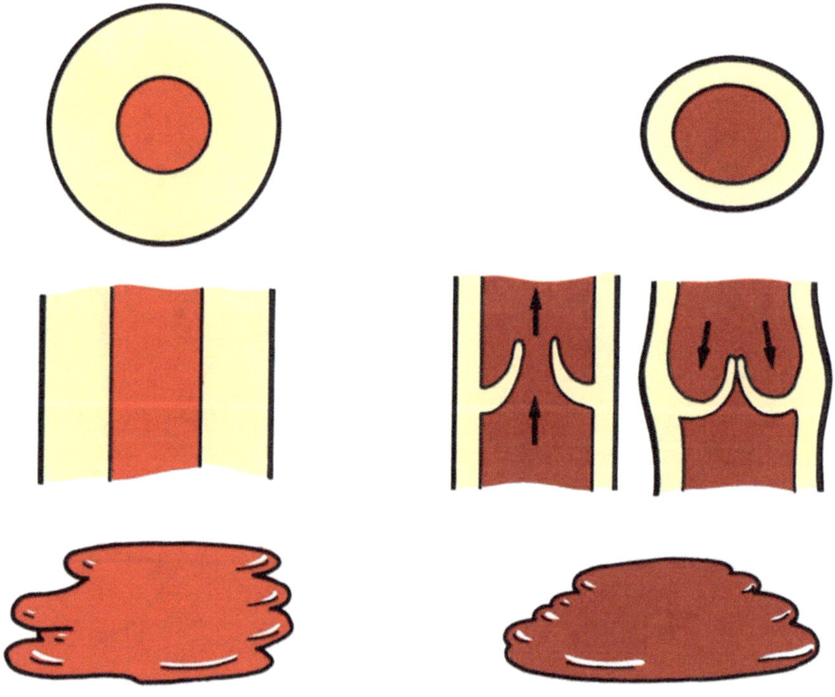

Figure 4.2 (a) Structure of artery and arterial blood. (b) Structure of vein and veinous blood.

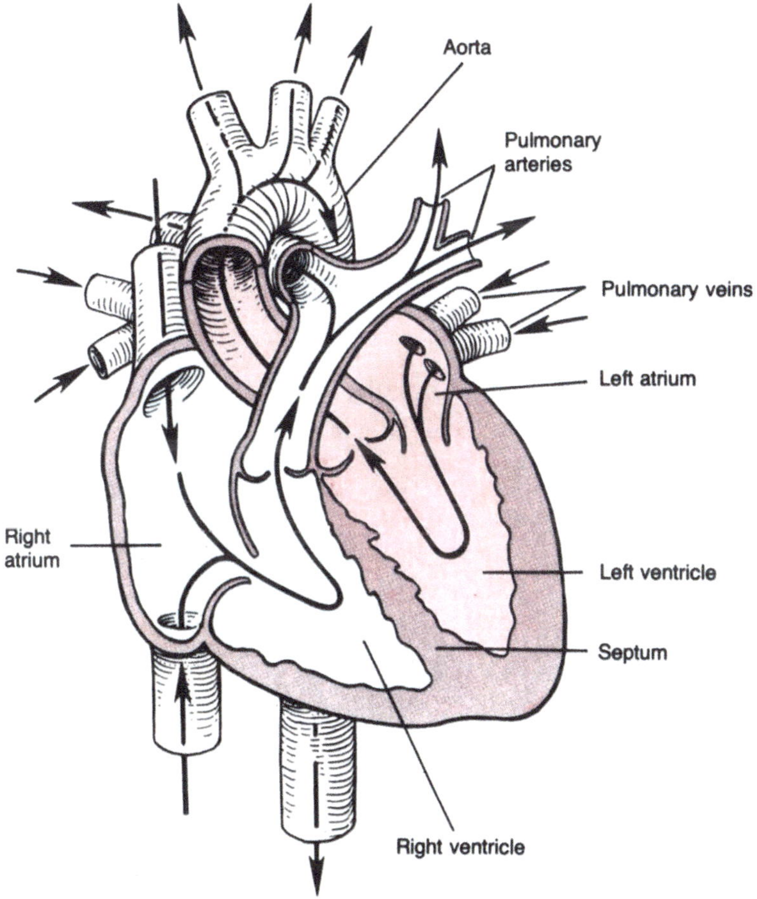

Figure 4.4 The heart

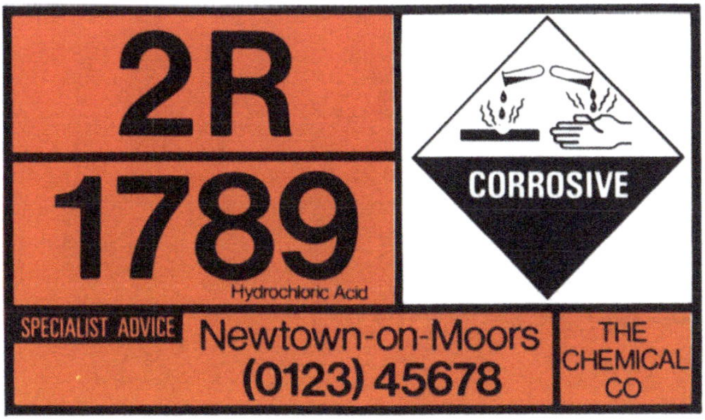

Figure 7.1 Hazard warning panel

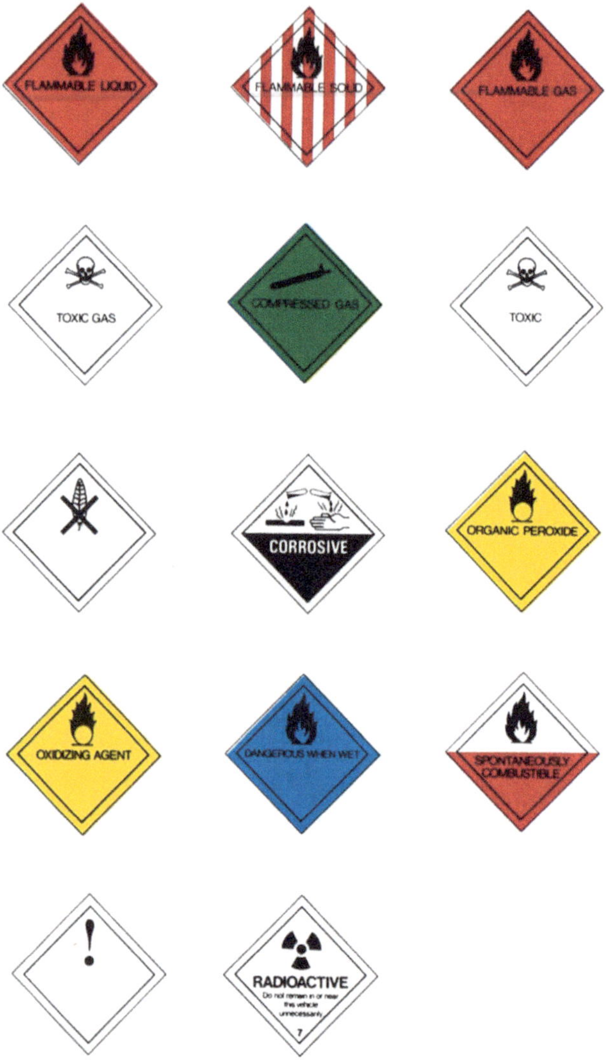

Figure 7.2 Symbols used for hazard warning

involving sensation or muscle activity in the head and neck.

The spinal cord occupies the vertebral canal in the vertebral column and is the elongated part of the central nervous system. It serves as a link between the brain and nerve supply to the trunk and limbs. The cord gives off 31 pairs of nerves at intervals along its length. Each nerve is concerned with sensation and muscle activity in parts of the body.

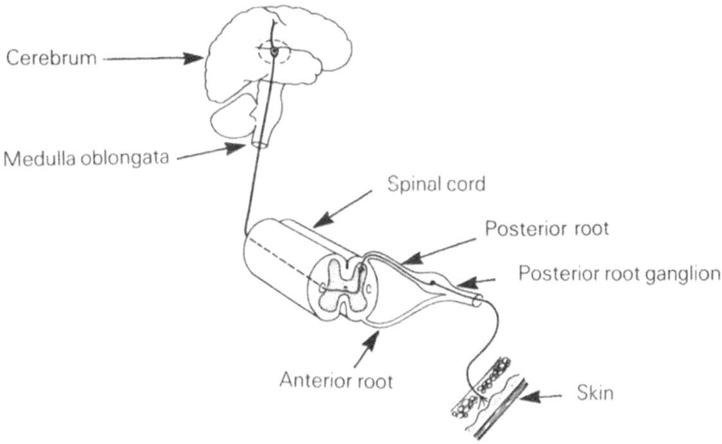

Figure 5.2 A stimulus applied to the skin produces an impulse which is registered in the sensory part of the brain

A stimulus of touch, pain, heat or cold applied to the skin produces an impulse which travels along the sensory nerve and spinal cord to be registered in the sensory part of the brain (Figure 5.2). If action is required by the body, the brain transmits a message from the motor section of the brain to the voluntary muscles involved. This impulse is transmitted down the spinal cord and along the motor nerve to the muscle (Figure 5.3).

Although the nerve impulse is transmitted very quickly, it can still take a long time to travel up and down the spinal cord. There may be a situation where a very quick response is required to a stimulus. On this occasion the sensory impulse enters the spinal cord but any further journey towards the brain is avoided and the impulse leaves the spinal cord at the same level, travelling along the motor nerve to the voluntary muscle involved. This is known

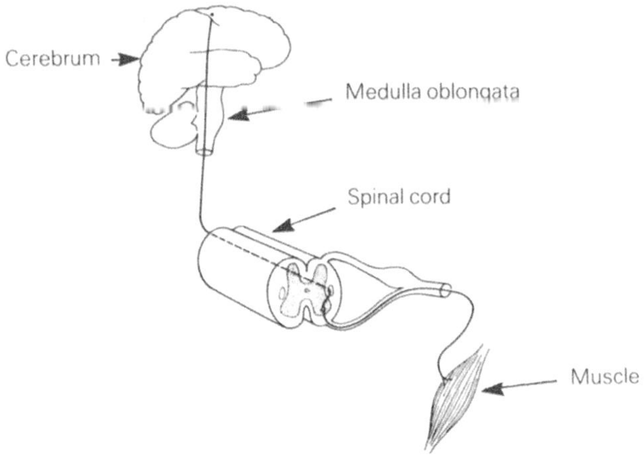

Figure 5.3 A message is transmitted from the motor section of the brain to the voluntary muscles

as a reflex arc. A typical reflex arc can be tested by gently hitting the knee below the kneecap with a patella hammer. This produces a reflex kicking action when the muscles are stimulated.

At any one point in the spinal cord there are nerve fibres being carried to and from the part of the body below that point. Damage to the spinal cord, as may be produced in a fracture of the spine, results in loss of sensation and muscle power in that part of the body supplied below the damaged area.

THE AUTONOMIC NERVOUS SYSTEM

The autonomic nervous system is a network of nerves which supply and regulate the internal organs, blood vessels and some glands (Figure 5.4). These structures, unlike the voluntary muscles, function without knowledge or effort.

The two components of the autonomic nervous system, the sympathetic and the parasympathetic systems, act in opposite ways to regulate the organs – one producing stimulation and the other producing relaxation.

Stimulation of the sympathetic system prepares the body for action in an emergency, by increasing the heart rate, decreasing bowel activity and relaxing the bladder.

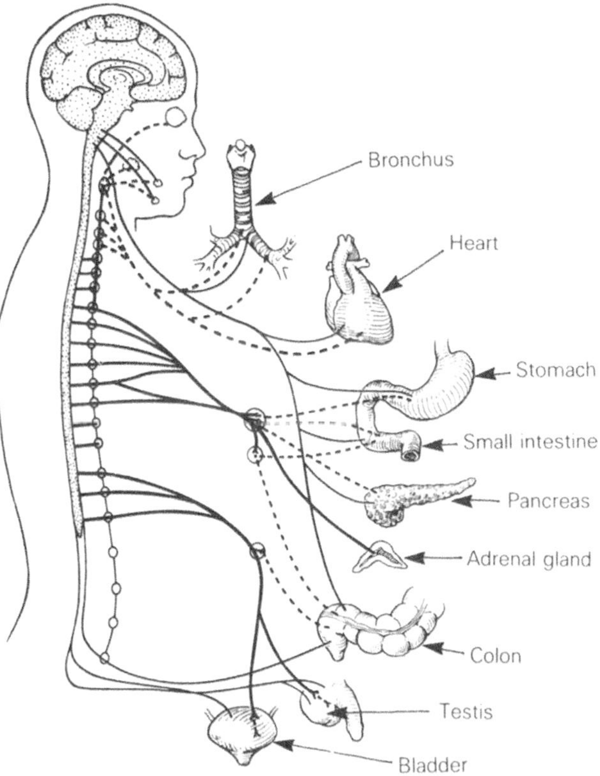

Figure 5.4 The autonomic nervous system

IMPAIRED CONSCIOUSNESS

A fully alert state requires an intact and functioning brain. Between the states of fully conscious and coma there are stages where the casualty is only partially conscious and has some, although incomplete, awareness of his surroundings.

Levels of consciousness

(1) Fully conscious – the casualty is aware of his surroundings and is able to answer questions normally.

(2) Drowsy – the casualty can be roused without difficulty and is

able to answer questions normally.

(3) Stupor – the casualty can be roused only with difficulty and the answers to questions are unreliable.

(4) Coma – the casualty cannot be roused, even with painful stimuli.

The division is not clear-cut and the levels of responsiveness are given as a guideline. There is a gradual transition from one level to the next and in practice it is better to record the casualty's answers to a few questions, so that, for example, it is known that half an hour ago he could give his name and address. Any deterioration in his condition would then be documented. This is particularly useful when handing the casualty over for further care.

The word 'coma' means 'deep sleep' and is the state of prolonged unconsciousness. It is caused by some disorder which acts generally on the nervous system.

Causes of unconsciousness

(1) Fainting,
(2) Infantile convulsions,
(3) Stroke,
(4) Head injury,
(5) Shock,
(6) Heart attack,
(7) Asphyxia,
(8) Poisoning,
(9) Epilepsy,
(10) Diabetes.

Fainting

A faint is a brief loss of consciousness resulting from a temporary reduction in the blood supply to the brain. It may be caused by fright, pain, an emotional reaction to bad news, exhaustion, lack of food, or physical inactivity – from the pooling of blood in the leg muscles.

There is usually some warning of an impending faint, with the casualty swaying and becoming unsteady. He is pale, sweating and develops impaired consciousness. If the faint develops, he becomes unconscious with a slow, weak pulse.

Infantile convulsions (febrile convulsions)

Any childhood illness, particularly throat and ear infections, may be associated with a high temperature and cause a convulsion. Despite the high temperature, mother's natural reaction with a sick child is to put a blanket around the child, to keep it warm. This increases the temperature and the risk of a convulsion.

If the child becomes very hot during an illness, every effort must be made to keep him cool. Excess clothing must be removed and the child sponged with tepid water to encourage heat loss by evaporation.

If a convulsion occurs, typical twitching movements of the muscles occur with the eyes rolling upwards. The airway must be protected and medical aid sought.

Stroke

A stroke is one of the commonest causes of coma and is caused by either a cerebral haemorrhage, where blood leaks from one of the blood vessels supplying the brain, or a cerebral thrombosis, where there is a clot in one of the blood vessels. The cause of the stroke may be associated with high blood pressure or hardening of the arteries.

Each part of the brain has a particular function and the extent of the stroke depends entirely on the extent of the disruption in the blood supply. It can vary from a temporary loss of function involving the power of speech, to long-term handicap when one side of the body is paralysed.

The casualty may complain of general ill-health during the hours or days preceding the stroke – but the onset of the stroke is always sudden. The blood vessels may be ruptured by physical effort or excitement, or this may occur during sleep. There may be a severe headache, or confusion and, unless the stroke is very mild, consciousness is lost within a few minutes.

The effect of the stroke is to produce paralysis or weakness on one side of the body with loss of bladder and bowel control.

A stroke may be rapidly fatal and emergency measures should

be considered, with protection of the casualty's airway. If the casualty is unconscious he should be placed in the recovery position. If he is conscious he should be placed in the most comfortable position until medical help arrives – with special care being taken with the airway, as the casualty may have lost the ability to swallow and saliva will accumulate in the mouth.

Head injury

Most head injuries are due to road traffic accidents or industrial accidents. Occasionally they are caused by a fall. There may be a scalp wound or damage to the skull, but, even in the absence of such damage, the most important consideration is the state of the brain rather than the state of the skull.

The scalp is well supplied with blood vessels and a scalp wound bleeds freely, causing some anxiety to the casualty. If the wound penetrates to the bone, there is a great danger that infection may spread to the bone. Any management of a scalp wound should therefore include assessment of the damage sustained, the presence of a foreign body and the level of consciousness.

Concussion

This is a condition resulting from a head injury when there is a general impairment of brain function. It is thought to be due to direct injury to nerve cells – as a result of a general 'shaking about' of the brain. It is reversible in milder cases.

The casualty may be confused and disorientated for a short time. He may be unconscious for a few seconds. Some mental functions may be affected for several hours – yet he can perform complicated activities in an automatic way and remember nothing about them afterwards. Post-, and pretraumatic amnesia may be alarming and vomiting may occur. A persistent headache may develop.

Compression

A severe blow to the head may cause compression on the brain, as a result of a depressed fracture or bleeding within the skull. If there is a large depressed fracture, the signs of compression will appear soon after the injury. If compression is caused by an increasing accumulation of blood clot within the skull, concussion usually appears first, followed by a characteristic lucid interval of one or more hours duration. The casualty then becomes confused and irritable with a deepening level of unconsciousness. The smell of alcohol on the breath may suggest that he is simply drunk and is in no particular danger.

He may start twitching and develop weakness or paralysis of the limbs on the side opposite to the head injury. On the side of the injury, the pupil contracts and then dilates – giving an important sign of unequal pupils. The temperature rises, the pulse falls and the breathing becomes noisy.

The diagnosis of compression injury to the brain is an emergency situation and the casualty must be transported to hospital immediately for appropriate treatment.

Epilepsy

In the 16th century epilepsy was described as the 'falling evil' and the nature of epilepsy was not discovered until 1929 when a method was devised of recording the electrical activity of the brain – an electroencephalogram. This showed that an epileptic convulsion or seizure was produced by a burst of excessive electrical activity from the brain. An epileptic is a person who is liable to suffer recurrent epileptic seizures.

The two main forms of epilepsy are:

(1) petit mal (absence seizures),
(2) grand mal.

Petit mal (absence seizures) Petit mal can begin at any time in children of school age. The attack or 'absence' begins without warning and there is a brief loss of consciousness lasting for a few seconds. The child stares with a rather dazed appearance. He may stop whatever activity he was doing – but there is no convulsion. The episode may be mistaken for day dreaming, but his eyes may flicker and he may be incontinent. As soon as the attack has finished, he carries on as though nothing has happened.

There may be several attacks each day and this could interfere with his school work. Drug treatment can control petit mal quite well, and an important aspect of management is the diagnosis and referral for treatment.

Grand mal A grand mal seizure is the dramatic form of epilepsy. It may begin with an aura, or warning. Depending on the site of the electrical activity in the brain, this may be either a strange taste, smell or an inability to speak. The electrical activity is associated with a generalized powerful muscular contraction – the tonic phase of the attack. The casualty loses consciousness and falls to the ground. The jaw muscles contract and the tongue may be bitten. The respiratory muscles go into spasm and breathing stops. The casualty becomes cyanosed. This phase lasts for up to 30 seconds.

The clonic phase follows and lasts for 2–3 minutes. During this phase the muscles contract and relax repeatedly, producing short, sharp, jerky movements. Foaming at the mouth, eyes rolling upwards and incontinence of urine may occur.

The casualty remains unconscious for a variable time and this is followed by a period of sleep or confusion.

Management of grand mal epilepsy As the epileptic attack may occur without warning, the casualty will usually be unconscious on the floor and convulsing before the first-aider is aware of the situation.

Any furniture within the reach of the casualty should be removed to prevent him hurting himself. He should be placed in the recovery position to allow secretions to drain out of the mouth, and his general condition should be observed and monitored until the convulsion has finished.

Particular care should be taken to ensure a good airway during the convulsion, but forcing open the mouth as a routine procedure should be avoided. Teeth may be broken in an attempt or the first-aider may get his fingers bitten! If a good airway can be maintained, there is no need for further intervention. If, however, there are signs of asphyxia caused by a blocked airway, every effort must be made to unblock the airway by removing dentures or lifting the tongue forward. Entry into the mouth should be between the stronger side teeth rather than the thinner front teeth – to reduce the possibility of damage to the teeth. Even this is a small price to pay if asphyxia and death during an epileptic fit can be prevented.

After the convulsion the casualty may enter a phase of postconvulsion automatism and wander around in a dazed state – unaware of his surroundings, or people talking to him.

Examination of the unconscious casualty

It is usually not immediately obvious why a casualty is unconscious. Any life-threatening situation must be discovered and corrected before proceeding further with the examination – as resuscitation may be required. The airway must be checked to make sure it is patent and the pulse must be checked, noting its rate and strength.

The casualty should be quickly examined for dampness, indicating severe bleeding, as this must be controlled.

The next step is to assess the depth of unconsciousness by finding out what response the casualty gives to a painful stimulus. The easiest way is to pinch the skin or rub the knuckles on the skin over the sternum. A comatose casualty will not respond at all, but a person who is less deeply unconscious may rouse, although he will be unaware of his surroundings or the events taking place.

Relatives or bystanders should be asked about the events leading up to the onset of unconsciousness and the length of time the casualty has been unconscious. Drugs, alcohol, poisons and previous illness may all be important as a cause of unconsciousness. The casualty may be wearing a Medical Information tag around his neck or wrist – or a diagnostic card (diabetic, steroid or anticoagulant) may be in his pocket or wallet.

The unconscious casualty should then be given a very detailed examination, as any part of the body may give the clue to the cause of the unconsciousness.

The skin

A pale, cold, clammy skin will indicate shock and further examination will be required to determine the cause of the shock.

Cyanosis will indicate an asphyxiating condition, and this may be associated with noisy breathing.

Carbon monoxide poisoning produces a cherry-red colour to the skin.

A very cold skin, with slow respiration and a slow pulse, may indicate hypothermia.

There may be evidence of trauma, producing severe haemorrhage, or scars of injections in diabetics and drug addicts

The breath

Smelling the casualty's breath may provide a clue. The characteristic smell of alcohol may be present, or the 'pear-drop' smell of diabetic coma.

The head

There may be contusions or lacerations on the scalp, suggesting the possibility of a fracture of the skull. The ears and nose should be examined for evidence of leakage of cerebrospinal fluid or blood. This would be a significant finding and indicate a fracture of the base of the skull.

A bitten tongue may be the only clue that an epileptic attack has just finished.

Corrosive burns on the lips and in the mouth would indicate poisoning. Dentures should be removed at this point, as they may cause a problem at any stage with the airway.

The pupils may be dilated in alcohol intoxication; pin-point in drug abuse; and unequal in head injury producing cerebral compression.

Central nervous system

The presence of convulsions, or even mild twitching, should be noted. The response to stimulation may differ on the two sides of the body. A painful stimulus may produce an instant movement of the arm or leg on one side, but no movement at all on the side paralysed by a stroke.

A sudden loss of consciousness associated with an emotional situation and a slow pulse may suggest syncope. In this case, unconsciousness is not usually deep or prolonged.

The rest of the body should be carefully examined for evidence of injury sustained in falling to the ground at the onset of unconsciousness. Evidence of dampness around the pelvis may indicate incontinence, as a consequence of an epileptic fit.

The unconscious casualty should not be moved unnecessarily. If he has to be moved to enable a proper examination to be carried out, he should be carefully rolled to one side – taking great care to move the body as a whole and not twist the spine. Help may be required from a colleague to maintain the casualty in this position until the examination is completed.

Recovery position

The reasons for the recovery position are to:

(1) maintain an open airway,
(2) prevent the inhalation of vomit and secretions,
(3) provide a stable position.

A casualty who is recovering from a state of unconsciousness is liable to vomit. This is a potentially serious hazard as the unconscious casualty is unable to protect his own airway. He must be placed in the recovery position with the head and neck in the extended position so that an open airway can be maintained. Secretions and vomit will then drain from the airway without being inhaled.

The position of the arms and legs provides a stable position for the casualty. Injuries to the arms and legs may prevent the standard positioning of the casualty. In this case, a rolled-up blanket placed behind the casualty can be used to maintain a stable position even when the arms and legs are extended.

The unconscious casualty should not be left on his own – even when he is in the recovery position, unless the situation makes this a practical impossibility.

Record keeping in brain injury

Accurate recording of observations is most important in the first-aid management of head injury. This is essential when an attempt is being made to recognize the presence of an early compression injury.

The observations and recording should include:

(1) the time of observations,
(2) the level of consciousness – which should include details of the casualty's ability to answer questions,
(3) the pulse,
(4) the size of the pupils.

If there is a long delay before the casualty reaches hospital and more than one first-aider is involved in recording details of the casualty, the actual observation record should be handed over to the person who takes over the next period of observation, so that a continuing record can be obtained.

6
Burns

Injuries from burns and scalds often result in tragic loss of life. The common cause, that of clothing catching fire, can produce devastating injuries in a few, frightening, minutes. The origin of the burns is 75% from domestic causes and 25% from industrial causes. Many of these burns, particularly the domestic burns, could be avoided if some thought was given to prevention.

Sources of danger

(1) Naked flames – coal fires, butane camping stoves, matches;
(2) Inflammable liquids – petrol, paraffin, paint 'thinners';
(3) Bonfires and fireworks;
(4) Hot fluids – teapot, saucepan, bath;
(5) Cooking appliances – frying pan, chip pan;
(6) Industrial – molten metal, chemical, friction, flames, electrical.

Butane camping stoves are an important source of danger because in daytime the flame is almost invisible. Burns from petrol and paraffin are increasing slightly because of the tendency to use this method as a means of suicide protest. The sale of fireworks is declining, but there is still a regular flow of injuries on Bonfire Night. Children should be protected from the danger of hot fluids in the house. A child may anticipate that the bath water is ready – only to find that the hot water has been put in first and the child becomes scalded.

The people at risk from burn injuries are:

(1) *Children* – who have yet to learn from experience that contact with hot objects produces pain and damage.

(2) *The elderly and frail* – who have forgotten what experience should have told them, or they may, in a moment of weak mobility, fall onto flames or stumble and knock over a saucepan of boiling liquid.

(3) *The handicapped* – who, through no fault of their own, find themselves in a situation where a burn injury is inevitable. The stroke patient may attempt to walk, but only succeeds in falling onto the fire. The epileptic patient may fall onto the fire during the course of an epileptic fit.

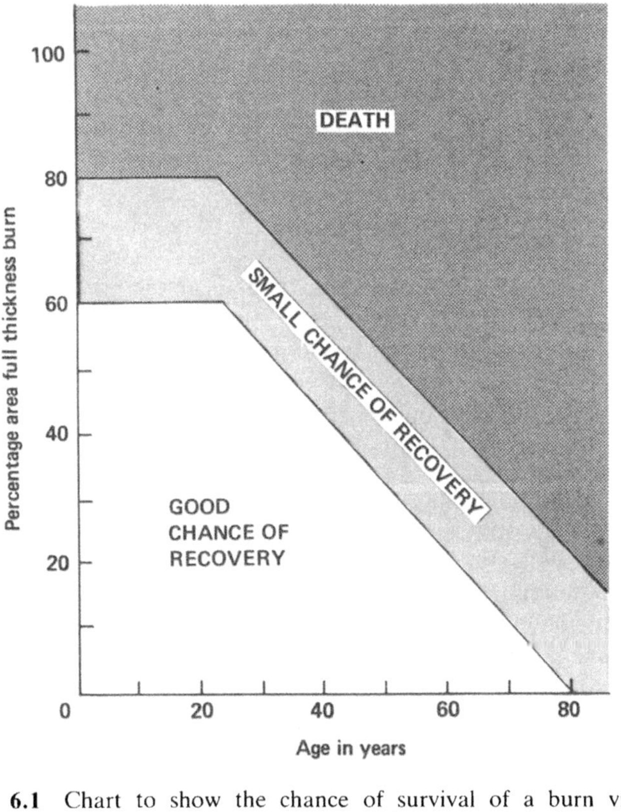

Figure 6.1 Chart to show the chance of survival of a burn victim depending on his age and the percentage surface area of the burn

The risk that is taken can be very great. It is possible to assess the chance of survival depending on the age of the casualty and the percentage surface area of the burn involved (Figure 6.1).

The Rule of 90 If the sum of the age of the casualty and the percentage surface area of the burn is more than 90 there is very little chance of survival.

COMPLICATIONS OF BURNS

(1) Shock,
(2) Infection,
(3) Local complications – sepsis, contractures.

Shock

The heat of the burn produces direct damage to the tissues involved, resulting in damage to the capillaries and an escape of plasma from the blood into the tissues. There can be a dramatic swelling of the tissues and blister formation if the skin is not broken. When the blisters burst, plasma leaks from the skin surface.

The loss of plasma from the circulation may be so great that the casualty is at risk of becoming shocked. However, the first-aider may be misled by the casualty's clinical condition by waiting for the common signs of shock to appear, namely a pale, cold, clammy skin. The skin is frequently not pale in the initial stages, and as the casualty has been burned, the skin is likely to be hot and dry, rather than cold and clammy!

The clue to the accurate clinical state is found in the amount of plasma producing blisters on the skin surface, or leaking as an exudate from the burn. This is directly related to the surface area of the burn, and the severity of the burn can be assessed by calculating the percentage of the surface area of the burn. The onset of shock can be forecast if the surface area of the burn is more than 15% in an adult, or more than 10% in a child.

The Rule of 9

The body is divided into areas of 9% and this can give a quick assessment of the surface area involved (Figure 6.2).

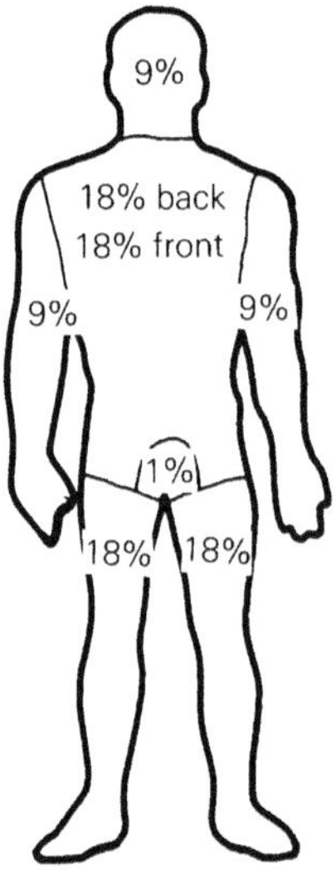

Figure 6.2 The rule of 9

If the casualty has scattered multiple burns, it is worth remembering that the surface area of the casualty's hand is approximately 1% of the total surface area. Therefore superimposing the surface area of the casualty's hand over each part of the scattered burn will give some guide to the total surface area of the burn (Figure 6.3).

Shock is aggravated by exposure to cold and severe pain – therefore inappropriate or careless handling of the casualty should be avoided. The appearance of shock is an indication of a deterioration in the casualty's condition, and it is hoped that by speedy removal to hospital, and plasma replacement in hospital, the serious consequences of shock may be avoided.

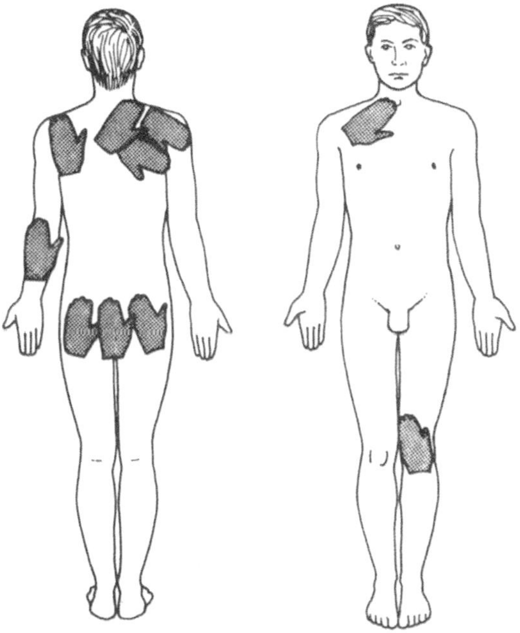

Figure 6.3 The casualty's hand is approximately 1% of the total surface area of his skin

Infection

Inappropriate or careless handling of the burn wound may result in infection, which may cause death within a few days from septicaemia (blood poisoning).

The burn wound is susceptible to any source of infection, whether it is self-infection from the patient, via nose or throat droplet spray, infection on the skin or clothes – or cross-infection from other people giving first aid. Any septic focus, contaminated hands, instruments or dressings, presents a source of danger to the casualty.

DEPTH OF BURN

The depth of damage to the skin (Figure 6.4) may be:

(1) Partial thickness
  (a) superficial
  (b) deep,
(2) Full thickness.

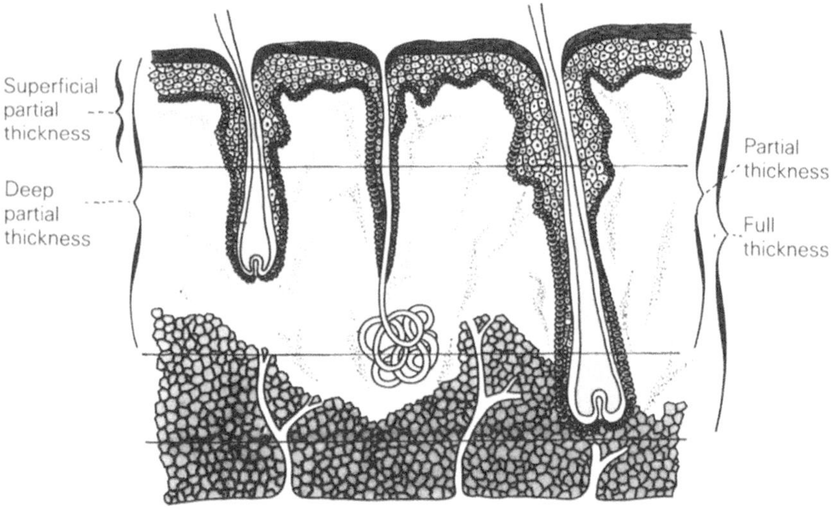

Figure 6.4 Section through the skin showing depth of skin associated with different severities of burn

The depth of the burn gives a further indication of the severity of a burn for treatment, and is related to the length of time the skin is in contact with the source of heat. It is of lesser importance in assessing the question of plasma loss and the development of shock compared with the measurement of the surface area of the burn.

Superficial burn

This occurs in sunburn and characteristically produces redness without the formation of blisters. It is very painful – as those who have endured sunburn will verify! Because the burn is superficial, the sweat glands and hair follicles are not destroyed and the skin is able to regenerate from the islands of epidermal cells surrounding these structures. Peeling takes place and there is no scarring.

Deep partial thickness (deep dermal) burn

The skin is destroyed down to the deeper layers and the burn produces blistering, or, if the skin surface is broken, an exudate. Regeneration of the skin is slower as, at this deeper level, there are fewer islands of epidermal cells.

Full thickness burn

The skin is destroyed down to the level of the subcutaneous fat. The skin has to grow in from the edges of the wound and a hard, dry black slough is produced in the healing process. Collagen fibres are laid down in the deep layers during the healing process and form a scar. They may contract and produce deformities.

This type of burn requires skin grafting at one or more stages in healing.

FIRST-AID MANAGEMENT

The major consideration in the management of a burn is to remove the source of damage in the skin – the heat. This is achieved by immersing the burn in cold water for at least 10 mins. A good indication of progress is that the pain from the burn wound gradually eases. If the pain returns, this is an indication that damage is continuing and the burn wound should be immersed in cold water again.

Great care should be taken to ensure that the burn wound does not become infected. A sterile, non-fluffy, dressing should be applied. The ideal dressing should be large enough to reach above and below the burn, and thick enough to prevent plasma soaking through to the outside of the dressing. If this happens the burn wound will be susceptible to airborne infection, which will land on the plasma-soaked dressing and travel through the dressing to the burn.

If rapid transfer of the casualty to hospital can be achieved, there is little more to be done in the first-aid management of a simple burn. However, if there are difficulties with transport, involving either long distances or time, and a lack of adequate first-aid supplies, some improvisation may be required – using clean, dry linen, etc. The burn casualty may also begin to complain of thirst, and this gives some indication of the loss of plasma. Some attempt can be made to replace the body fluid by giving the casualty frequent sips of water. The amount should not exceed one glass per hour because an excessive intake of water may make the casualty vomit – adding to the problems of management.

Clothing on fire

This remains a frequent cause of domestic burn – despite the attempts at accident prevention. The casualty becomes panic stricken and runs around in an attempt to escape the flames. The result is simply to fan the flames and allow them to become more vigorous. While the casualty remains in the upright position the flames will move steadily towards the head and airway. Quick action is required from the first-aider to bring the casualty to the ground and smother the flames by wrapping a blanket round the casualty. If this is not possible, the flames can be doused with water using whatever method is immediately available.

Once the flames are out, the burnt clothing is sterile and there is no immediate need to remove it. There is a danger that any attempt to remove clothing may also remove skin adherent to it.

Burns to the head

A burn to the face involving the mouth and nose can cause a problem if resuscitation is required. A burn to the eye may result in loss of sight, or the swollen eyelids will temporarily interfere with vision and give the casualty the impression that he is blind.

Burns to the hand

The fingers are difficult to bandage and it may be appropriate to cover the hand by putting it in a clean polythene bag to prevent infection reaching the burn surface during the journey to hospital.

Electrical burns

Electricity will cause a burn if the voltage and current are high enough. The electrical shock may have stopped the casualty's heart and lungs working, but the current must be switched off before resuscitation is attempted. This is particularly important in incidents involving high voltage electricity pylons. Despite the overwhelming desire to assist the casualty, the first aider must not approach within 20 yards of the pylon until officially told that the electricity supply has been switched off. This may involve a delay of half an hour or more.

Electrical burns characteristically produce a burn at both the entry and exit points. Although the apparent damage may be quite small, as indicated by the area of skin involved, the damage to the deeper tissues can be very extensive – sometimes resulting in amputation of a limb.

Lightning

Depending on the intensity of the lightning strike, the burn may have a leaf or fern-like appearance. A major lightning strike produces a severe burn at the point of contact and exit – usually through one foot as the lightning 'earths'.

Chemical burns

Chemical burns may be caused by a large variety of chemicals used in the home, in industry and during war.

The chemical should be removed from the affected area by thoroughly flooding the skin with water or the antidote, if one exists and is readily available. If the incident occurs in a factory where chemicals are used routinely, there may be instructions to be followed in the event of a chemical burn. If provided, protective clothing should be worn – but speed is essential and precious time should not be wasted in a fruitless search for protective clothing and the antidote, when the burn could be dealt with by thorough flooding with water, and arrangements made for the speedy transfer of the casualty to hospital.

A chemical burn to the eye should be dealt with in the same way – thorough flooding or irrigation of the eye with water, to ensure that all remnants of the chemical are washed away. Care must be taken if the chemical is lime because lime reacts with water and the result of the chemical process is to produce heat – thereby aggravating the chemical burn. Obviously it is very difficult to remove *all* traces of lime, but the large particles of lime must be removed before flooding the eye thoroughly with water.

An eye pad and bandage should be applied and the casualty transferred to hospital.

Friction burns

Friction burns are produced when the skin is in contact with a moving surface. The extent of the damage to the tissues varies from the superficial burn and discolouration caused by a rope burn, to damage to the deeper tissues, including tendons, when prolonged contact occurs with a rough surface, such as an electric floor polisher.

Referral for medical advice or treatment will naturally depend on the extent of the injury.

Rescue of the burned casualty

The victim *in a burning room* may be unconscious and asphyxiating from smoke inhalation. He must be removed quickly from the area and expert help may be available from specially trained personnel with proper protective equipment and breathing apparatus.

The victim with *clothes on fire* should be put on the floor and the flames smothered, or the flames doused with water. Clothing that has been on fire is sterile and need not be removed during the journey to hospital.

The victim *scalded with hot fluids or chemicals* should be doused with copious water. Remnants of the chemicals will remain on the clothing and continue to damage the skin. The clothing must be removed to prevent the continuing damage.

THE BATTERED CHILD

If the casualty is a child, the first-aider should be alert to the possibility that the burn, bruise, wound or fracture may indicate a non-accidental injury – and that the first-aider may be the person of first contact in a battered baby incident.

Suspicious burns are the small round burns caused by lighted cigarettes; burns with a straight edge – which may indicate branding; burns involving the buttocks and genitalia – caused by dunking the child in a hot bath; and whether the circumstances of the burn correlate with the appearance of the burn (for example, a multiple scattered burn that is blamed on the hot water bottle bursting in bed should rouse some suspicion).

Any suspicion should be conveyed to the appropriate authorities, the child's Health Visitor, Social Services, the GP, the police or the local Casualty Department. Circumstances will usually dictate that the child be taken to hospital for treatment, and this is regarded as a 'place of safety' for the child.

7 Poisoning

Acute poisoning is an urgent medical problem, and is usually caused by a self-administered overdose of drugs. Of the 130 000 cases of self-poisoning each year, more than 3000 result in death. Recent research and development in the pharmaceutical industry has produced new sleeping tablets and antidepressant drugs with an emphasis on safety, and these are less likely to cause death in an overdose. An attempt has been made to reduce the risk of children poisoning themselves, by producing tablet bottles with safety tops fitted. Despite this, poisoning in children remains a frequent problem.

Many people who intentionally poison themselves do not intentionally seek to kill themselves. It is frequently no more than a gesture and a cry for help. Unfortunately things can go wrong, and, owing to mistaken timing or dosage, that cry for help can result in death.

Poisoning may be:

(1) accidental,
(2) intentional,
(3) homicidal – it is worth bearing this aspect in mind and taking care not to leave fingerprints on tablet bottles etc. when dealing with poisoning – in case you become the prime suspect!

Poisons can enter the body through:

(1) the mouth,
(2) the lungs,

(3) injection – insect and snake bites, drugs of addiction,
(4) absorption through the skin – pesticides.

GENERAL MANAGEMENT OF POISONING

Successful emergency treatment of acute poisoning depends on a combination of speed and common sense, as well as recognition of the type of poison, the amount taken and the time since it was taken. Immediate action with resuscitation, if required, and urgent transport to hospital are the important aspects of first-aid management if there is to be any hope of achieving a satisfactory outcome.

Initial assessment

An initial assessment should determine the following:

(1) the presence of a heart beat,
(2) the presence of adequate respiration
  – is there a good airway?
  – is there cyanosis?
(3) the level of consciousness,
(4) the presence of convulsions,
(5) the temperature – hypothermia may occur and the patient will need to be kept warm.

First-aid management

(1) Maintain a clear airway. Dentures and vomit should be removed and the casualty's airway should be supervised. Artificial respiration may be required but the mouth-to-mouth method must not be used if the poison is corrosive. If the casualty is breathing normally, he should be placed in the recovery position to protect the airway.

(2) Monitor the heart rate. External cardiac compression will be required if the heart stops.

(3) Identify the poison. If there is difficulty identifying the poison, any tablets or bottles found near the casualty should be noted and arrangements made for them to be taken to

hospital with the casualty. Any accompanying instruction leaflet should also be sent. If the poison is a gas, the casualty should be removed to fresh air as quickly as possible.

(4) Urgent transport to hospital. All cases of poisoning should be sent to hospital – even before symptoms of poisoning occur. Some poisons have a delayed action and early treatment will improve the chances of recovery.

The airway, respiration rate and heart rate should be monitored continually during transport to hospital – and resuscitation started if necessary. If the casualty vomits, the vomit should be kept, labelled and sent with the casualty to hospital.

If the journey to hospital involves travelling for several hours or if transport is not immediately available, an attempt should be made to reduce the effect of the poison in the body.

An important distinction must be made between non-corrosive and corrosive poisons.

Non-corrosive poisons are tablets, liquid medicines and berries. It is worthwhile encouraging the casualty to vomit if it is less than 4 hours since the non-corrosive poison was taken. Aspirin compounds and some anti-depressant drugs cause a delay in stomach emptying and may remain in the stomach for up to 12 hours.

Do not attempt to induce vomiting by using salt solutions. These alter the body chemistry and this may have fatal consequences.

Do not attempt to make an unconscious casualty vomit. The unconscious casualty is unable to protect his airway and there is a danger that the vomit may block the airway or be inhaled.

Corrosive poisons are bleach, disinfectants, descalers, certain chemicals, dishwasher detergents and drain cleaners. A poison with a corrosive action can be identified by the burns it produces around the lips and chin. The corrosive effect continues down the oesophagus and into the stomach. If the casualty is encouraged to vomit, the corrosive effect will be repeated in the oesophagus as the poison is vomited. The corrosive poison, therefore, needs to be diluted by giving the casualty large quantities of water or milk.

The effect of the corrosive on the skin can be reduced by washing the area with plenty of water – taking care not to allow the water to enter the airway.

POISONING THROUGH THE MOUTH

The drugs most frequently taken are antidepressants, tranquillizers, sleeping tablets and pain-killing tablets. They may produce (Table 7.1):

(1) unconsciousness,
(2) reduced respiration rate,
(3) reduced cardiac function,
(4) convulsions.

Table 7.1 Features of drug overdose

	Skin	*Convulsions*	*Respiration*
Antidepressants	moist, warm	present	increased
Aspirin	dry, warm	present	depressed
Barbiturates	moist, cold, rash	absent	depressed
Paracetamol	pale	absent	normal

Alcohol

Large quantities of alcohol produce a state of inebriation, mental confusion and a lack of co-ordination of movement. An increase in blood flow through the skin produces a feeling of warmth. This also increases heat loss from the body – which could be a disadvantage if the person is going to be out in the cold for a long time, or stranded in snow.

The casualty may smell of alcohol, have a flushed appearance, be breathing heavily and start vomiting. The pupils may be dilated and he may become unconscious, leading to respiratory depression, coma and death.

The general effect of alcohol is depressant. The initial stimulant effect is due to a removal of inhibitions.

Methylated spirits is sometimes taken as a cheap

alternative to alcohol (ethanol). It produces abdominal pain, headache, muscle cramps, disturbance of vision with blindness, and convulsions.

Antifreeze (ethylene glycol) may produce similar signs to alcohol poisoning – without the smell of alcohol on the breath. If antifreeze is splashed into the eye it can produce an intense irritation, and requires flushing out with a copious flow of water.

Aspirin (salicylate) poisoning

Aspirin tablets continue to be a common source of accidental poisoning, particularly among children, who mistake the tablets for sweets. The most toxic form occurs from swallowing certain liniments containing methyl salicylate (oil of wintergreen) and death can result from a child swallowing one or two teaspoonsful.

The initial symptoms are vomiting, overbreathing, overactivity, and an increase in temperature. This leads to difficulty in breathing, lethargy, buzzing in the ears and, eventually, collapse, coma and death.

Antidepressants

This group of drugs presents a high risk in the overdose situation. They produce blurred vision, dry mouth, increased pulse, restlessness, convulsions and coma. An irregular pulse may develop, with cardiac arrest. An overdose must always be considered in a lonely person who is being treated for depression. The pharmaceutical companies are attempting to reduce the risk by developing new antidepressant drugs which have a much lower risk when an overdose is taken.

Barbiturates

Barbiturate poisoning is becoming less frequent as the frequency of prescribing this drug gets less. However, other sedative drugs are taking their place and cause similar problems in an overdose.

When barbiturates are taken in a suicide attempt, alcohol is often taken at the same time. This increases the duration of effect and the risk of death.

The casualty becomes unsteady with slurred speech, and

confusion. Coma develops leading to respiratory depression and death. In about 10% of cases, a rash develops.

Iron tablets

Iron tablets are frequently prescribed during pregnancy, and to treat anaemia. They are often very attractive to children, because of their colour, and are mistaken for sweets. However, they are extremely toxic to children and can quickly cause death.

Shortly after swallowing iron tablets, the casualty develops abdominal pain, vomiting and diarrhoea with blood. Coma and death occur within 6–8 hours in 20% of untreated cases. Some casualties show an initial improvement but may lapse into coma, with convulsions and death occurring within 24 hours.

Any suspected overdose of iron tablets must be referred to hospital urgently – even if there is doubt about the number of tablets the child may have taken.

Paraffin

Petroleum hydrocarbons (paraffin and petrol) are responsible for many cases of poisoning in children, through accidental swallowing. The child may complain of a burning sensation in the mouth, throat and stomach – from its irritant effect. This may produce coughing and a choking feeling. Lethargy and coma may follow.

The casualty is in danger of suffering damage to the lungs if paraffin is inhaled during vomiting. No attempt should be made, therefore, to make the casualty vomit.

Contaminated clothing should be removed quickly and any paraffin on the skin should be washed off. The casualty should be given milk to dilute the paraffin, and transferred to hospital urgently.

Paracetamol

An overdose of 30 tablets may cause severe liver damage, which will become apparent a few days later. There are few symptoms and signs associated with paracetamol overdose – apart from nausea and vomiting. Speedy removal to hospital is especially important, because a specific antidote may result in recovery if given within 10 hours of the overdose.

Paraquat

Paraquat is a weed-killer and is available in two forms. The liquid form contains 20% paraquat and is available to farmers for agricultural or industrial use. A granular preparation is available for the home gardener and contains 2.5% paraquat.

Splashing paraquat in the eyes leads to severe inflammation. Immediate irrigation with a copious flow of water is required and referral to hospital.

Paraquat on the skin produces inflammation and irritation, occasionally producing blisters. Some paraquat may be absorbed through the skin if contaminated clothing remains in contact with the skin for long periods. All contaminated clothing must therefore be removed and the splashes on the skin washed off.

Serious difficulties occur when paraquat is accidentally swallowed. This can occur unintentionally if the paraquat is stored in an inappropriate bottle – a pop bottle, which a child can find in a garage or greenhouse.

The immediate effects are produced by an irritant action and are nausea, vomiting and diarrhoea, with soreness of the mouth and difficulty in swallowing. Damage to most major organs occurs and is accompanied by convulsions, coma and death, which may occur within 48 hours.

If paraquat has been swallowed recently, vomiting should be induced quickly – if it has not already occurred. However, if treatment is started several hours after swallowing paraquat, vomiting should *not* be induced, as ulceration of the oesophagus may have occurred.

Speedy transfer to hospital for stomach washout is required.

Poisonous plants

Deadly nightshade produces cherry-sized berries which may be mistaken by children and adults for blueberries. They contain atropine, which produces a dry mouth, hot dry skin, blurred vision, restlessness, an increase in heart rate, and dilated pupils. The alternative name of 'belladonna' means 'beautiful lady' and refers to the once fashionable practice by ladies of putting an extract of deadly nightshade into their eyes to dilate the pupils – in the belief that this would make them appear more attractive.

Laburnum trees produce 'pea-pods' in the summer and children mistake these for an edible vegetable. The seeds contain cytisine, which produces abdominal pain, vomiting and dizziness.

Death cap mushroom (Amanita phalloides) is a well-known cause of mushroom poisoning but any non-edible mushroom may produce poisoning. The usual symptoms are violent abdominal colic, nausea, vomiting and diarrhoea. The symptoms occur about 1–2 hours after eating the poisonous mushrooms and may lead to dehydration.

POISONS THROUGH THE LUNGS

Carbon monoxide

Carbon monoxide poisoning may result from inhaling the fumes from a car exhaust, from coal-mine explosions or from coal or coke fires in a poorly ventilated room.

Carbon monoxide is odourless. The toxic effect is due to the greater affinity haemoglobin has for carbon monoxide than for oxygen, which is displaced by the carbon monoxide from haemoglobin – thus reducing the oxygen-carrying capacity of blood. A compound, carboxyhaemoglobin, is formed which is unable to carry oxygen and asphyxia is produced.

The level of toxicity depends on the length of exposure to the gas and the amount of carboxyhaemoglobin formed in the blood. Mild toxicity is associated with nausea, headache and dizziness. Increasing levels of carbon monoxide poisoning produce weakness, coma and death.

Carboxyhaemoglobin has a characteristic cherry-pink colour and this may be seen in the nail beds and lips. It will be more evident at postmortem.

The casualty should be dragged out of the contaminated environment and given assisted respiration. 100% oxygen should be given as soon as it is available.

North sea gas

North sea gas reduced the number of deaths resulting from inhalation of the domestic gas supply. However, poisoning can still occur as a result of a faulty burner, giving an incomplete combustion of gas, or poorly ventilated rooms.

Ammonia gas

Some refrigerators use ammonia in the cooling system. If a leak develops in the system, there will be an accidental exposure to ammonia fumes.

Ammonia is intensely irritating to the eyes and respiratory tract. Coughing and choking develop rapidly and can be quite alarming. Treatment involves removal of the casualty from the environment, and flushing the eyes with a copious supply of water.

Glue sniffing (solvent abuse)

In 1982 there were over 60 deaths from solvent abuse. Many different types of product are used, including glue, aerosol propellants, polystyrene cement, lighter refills and petrol. The most widely recognized are the highly volatile glues.

Despite the term 'glue sniffing', the effects of these products are achieved by deep inhalation. Small quantities are either bagged (put into a plastic bag and the contents inhaled) or huffed (put onto a cloth held near the mouth). A method giving great cause for concern is that of spraying a butane spray up the nose or in the mouth. The aerosol propellant is harmful and can cause death.

The immediate effect of glue sniffing is to produce a drunken behaviour with euphoria and hallucinations. The resulting irresponsible behaviour may result in a chargeable offence being committed – which may bring glue sniffers to the notice of the police.

Glue sniffing is suggested by the rather odd behaviour of the sniffer. He tends to be secretive about his activities. He develops a loss of appetite and general irritability – and his breath or clothing smell of solvent.

The long-term effect has yet to be established, although it is recognized that repeated glue sniffing may result in some brain damage within 1 year. Liver and kidney damage may also occur.

The circumstances in which the casualty is found usually indicate the diagnosis if first-aid measures are required. If the casualty is unconscious, he should be placed in the recovery position to protect his airway.

The important aspect is prevention, by educating teenagers about the hazards of glue sniffing.

POISONS INJECTED THROUGH THE SKIN

Insect stings and bites

A bee sting produces a sudden, intense, local pain with swelling and irritation. Some people become sensitized to bee venom and suffer increasingly severe reaction to successive bee stings. This may result in an anaphylactic reaction with a generalized rash, wheezing and death. Bee-keepers are stung most days and seem to develop a resistance to the effects of bee venom.

When the sting occurs, the barbed sting is usually left in the skin. It must be removed quickly because the venom sac continues to pump venom into the skin. It must not be grasped by the venom sac as this will squeeze further venom into the skin. The sting should be held with tweezers and pulled out of the skin. If tweezers are not available, the sting should be scraped off the skin with a finger nail.

Wasps and ants may produce similar distressing symptoms.

The pain and swelling produced by bites and stings may be relieved by a cold compress or calamine lotion.

Snake bites

Travellers to any part of the world may be at risk from snakes, which can be particularly hazardous, although acute poisoning due to venomous snakes is unusual in this country. The only venomous snake native to Britain is the adder. More exotic and unusual examples are kept in zoos, or at home in the care of enthusiastic amateurs.

A snake bite causes local pain and swelling. Other symptoms include vomiting and diarrhoea, abdominal colic and agitation.

The aim of treatment is to reduce the absorption of venom.

Various heroic forms of treatment have been discarded. Arterial tourniquets are painful, potentially dangerous and have no place in the first-aid management of snake bites. Incision of the area of the snake bite is also dangerous, as the underlying tendons and blood vessels may be damaged. Freezing the area involved simply provides the casualty with two problems – the snake bite and cold injury to the skin.

The bite should be washed thoroughly with soap and water. 95% of snake bites occur on limbs, and recent research has shown that a pressure bandage applied properly and comfortably over the site of the snake bite, combined with immobilization of the limb, reduces the rate of venom absorption. The bandage may be left in place for several hours, although a regular check should be made to make sure that the blood supply to the limb is not restricted. Care must be taken if the bite is on the trunk to ensure that the pressure bandage does not impede respiration. No attempt should be made to apply a pressure bandage to a snake bite on the neck!

Drugs of addiction

Narcotic drug abuse is becoming an increasing problem – particularly among teenagers who regard narcotics as another area of curiosity, and experiment with various drugs. For some the experiment leads to addiction, with all the associated personal health problems and social difficulties.

Cocaine is derived from the leaves of the South American coca tree. Local inhabitants chew the leaves to produce a feeling of relief from tiredness and hunger. Addicts take cocaine by injecting it into a vein, or as a snuff, which may cause ulceration inside the nose.

An overdose causes cerebral stimulation, with excitement and convulsions. The pupils become dilated and there is a sensation of ants crawling under the skin.

Heroin produces a strong dependence on the drug – resulting in an overwhelming desire to continue taking it, and a compulsion to obtain it by any means. If the drug is not taken, severe withdrawal symptoms occur. To avoid these the addict spends all his time and money on obtaining further supplies, and tends to neglect himself.

An overdose causes warm, sweating skin, pin-point pupils, a reduced depth and rate of respiration (to 6–10 breaths per minute) and unconsciousness. There may be evidence of abuse, with injection marks on the arms and legs.

Withdrawal symptoms usually begin at about the time of the next expected dose and include restlessness, yawning, sweating, abdominal pain, nausea, muscle twitching, 'gooseflesh' and spontaneous muscle spasms making the addict give kicking movements (known as 'kicking the habit').

Morphine produces similar effects.

Narcotic drugs in overdose produce unconsciousness. The first-aid management consists of support, with monitoring of the heart, airway and breathing – and transfer to hospital.

POISONING BY ABSORPTION THROUGH THE SKIN

Pesticides

The number of chemicals used to combat weeds and diseases in agriculture is increasing. Some are poisonous. If a person using pesticides becomes ill, all contaminated protective clothing should be removed with care, to avoid contamination of the first-aider. Any contaminated skin should be washed with soap and water. If pesticide has splashed into the eye, irrigation with a copious supply of water should be performed. The eye should then be covered with an eye pad and bandage.

The most widely used pesticides are the organophosphorus compounds and these vary in toxicity from low (malathion) to high (parathion). Symptoms include pinpoint pupils, slow pulse, abdominal pain, nausea, a tight feeling in the chest, shortness of breath with wheezing and sweating.

The casualty should be transported quickly to hospital, in the recovery position to ensure that the airway is kept clear. The heart and breathing should be monitored and resuscitation given if necessary.

The hospital should be informed about the name of the pesticide and any label or leaflet about the pesticide should accompany the casualty to hospital.

THE HAZCHEM (EMERGENCY ACTION) CODE

Hazardous substances are being transported more frequently by road and rail. When an accident involves leakage or spillage of a dangerous substance, it is imperative that the substance should be identified as soon as possible.

Dangerous substances can produce:

(1) radiation hazard,
(2) chemical hazard,
(3) biological hazard.

The Hazchem code indicates to the first person to arrive at the incident the initial action to be taken to minimize the danger to the public. The immediate action can be taken without detailed knowledge of the exact nature of the dangerous substance.

Hazard warning panels are displayed on transport vehicles in three positions – one on the back of the vehicle, and one on each side, as near to the front as possible (Figure 7.1). The panel is divided into four sections displaying:

(1) the diamond label hazard symbol (Figure 7.2),
(2) the Hazchem code using one number and one letter, with an additional letter E when appropriate,
(3) the United Nations identification number for the dangerous substance,
(4) a telephone number for specialist advice

The diamond label hazard symbol is one of a series of internationally agreed labels to give an easily understood warning of the nature of the hazard.

The code (Figure 7.3) is:

1 = water jets
2 = water, fog or spray
3 = foam
4 = dry agents

Any medium with a higher number than the one given in the Hazchem code may be used to deal with the dangerous substance, but under no circumstances should one with a lower number be used.

The first letter of the code forms part of PRSTWXYZ giving information on how to deal with spillage, and also information regarding personal protection (Figure 7.3). The first four letters PRST indicate substances which can be safely diluted with copious supplies of water and allowed to escape into drains. The letters WXYZ indicate substances which should be contained until further assistance can be provided.

The first and third pairs of letters PR and WX are used when full protection is required. The second and fourth pairs of letters ST and YZ indicate that breathing apparatus must be worn.

The alternate letters of the scale, P,S,W and Y, are used for substances which are potentially explosive.

The letter E appearing after the first letter indicates that evacuation should be considered as there is a high risk from either toxicity or explosion.

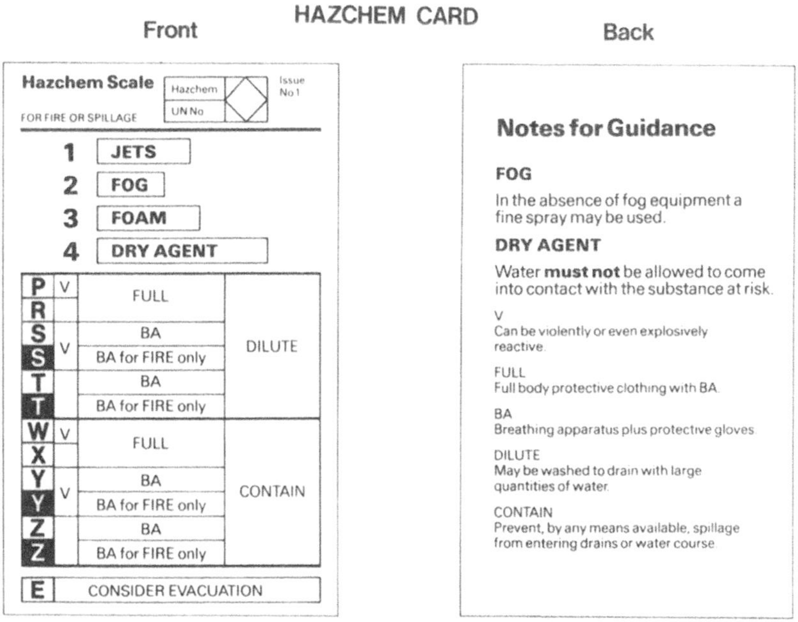

Figure 7.3 The Hazchem code

Tremcards

The TRansport EMergency card system gives additional information for the driver in an emergency incident, including details of first-aid management. This additional supply of information may be particularly useful when the driver of the vehicle has been injured in the accident and is not able to help with details of management.

8
Diabetes

Diabetes mellitus is a condition where the blood sugar is persistently raised. About 1% of the population are affected. Half of these remain undetected and are unaware of the fact, but 30 000 new cases of diabetes are detected each year. The condition may appear at any age, but the majority of cases occur after the age of 50.

PHYSIOLOGY OF DIABETES

Carbohydrates are metabolized in the stomach and intestine, and glucose is absorbed. Some glucose is stored in the liver until required, some is metabolized to provide energy and some is kept available in the circulating plasma and tissue fluids, ready to be taken up by the tissue cells in moments of additional energy requirements.

If the blood sugar rises above a certain level, sugar appears in the urine. To counter the rise in the blood sugar, insulin, which is a hormone released by the pancreas, increases the uptake of glucose by the tissue cells. Any interference with the production of insulin in the pancreas, or its effects on the uptake by the tissue cells, will upset the balance, increase the blood sugar level and produce a diabetic state.

THE EFFECTS OF DIABETES

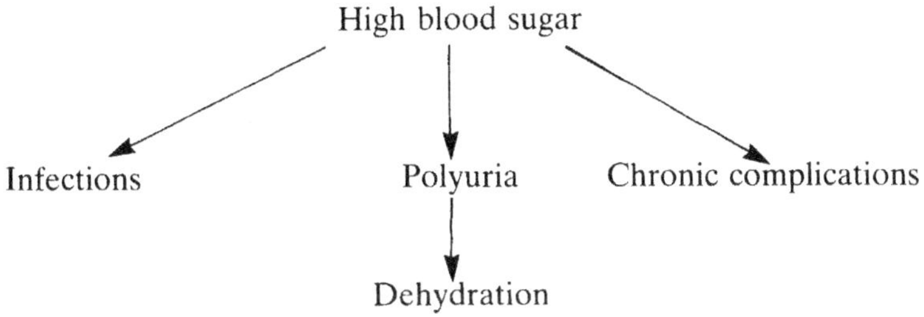

When the blood sugar level is high, sugar appears in the urine and more water is excreted by the kidneys (polyuria). The volume of urine may increase to 7–10 litres/day, producing an intense thirst. If the polyuria persists, there will eventually be signs of dehydration.

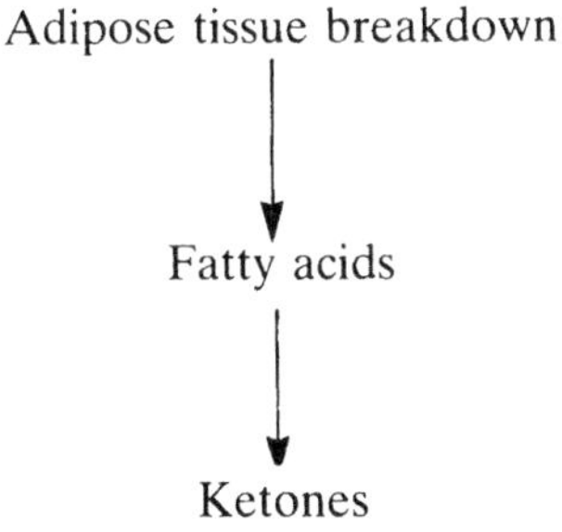

If the carbohydrate intake is not available to the body as a source of energy, tiredness will be produced. The body attempts to satisfy its energy requirements from other sources and breakdown of fat and protein occurs. The breakdown of fat results in the formation of ketones and these can be detected by the acetone smell on the breath. The metabolism of body protein to provide energy leads to weakness and weight loss.

The long-term problems of diabetes are related to infections of the skin, lungs and kidneys, together with cataract formation in the eyes and circulation problems leading to skin ulcers and gangrene.

TYPES OF DIABETES

Juvenile onset

This affects children and adults up to about 40 years old. There is a rapid onset of symptoms – thirst, polyuria, loss of weight and tiredness. In this group the pancreas fails to produce insulin for reasons which are, as yet, unclear (possibly caused by a virus infection). This type of diabetes therefore requires treatment with insulin injections and is also known as Insulin Dependent Diabetes Mellitus (IDDM).

Maturity onset

This affects middle-aged or elderly patients. They are often overweight and there is a slow onset of symptoms. It is less severe than the juvenile-onset type and can usually be controlled by means of diet or tablets. It is therefore known as Non-Insulin Dependent Diabetes Mellitus (NIDDM).

The diabetic on insulin injections is in a state of fine balance. The amount of insulin must be measured accurately to prevent the blood sugar rising out of control, and consideration must be given to the amount and type of food eaten – to balance the insulin received.

Various circumstances will upset the balance – an unexpected delay in getting a meal, prolonged exercise or an illness.

The diabetic is always potentially liable to lose control of his diabetic state and this may result in a *low* blood sugar (hypoglycaemia) or *high* blood sugar (hyperglycaemia).

HYPOGLYCAEMIA

The casualty may have been subjected to unexpected exercise, a missed meal or an overdose of insulin. Symptoms develop rapidly and include a feeling of weakness, sweating, palpitations, faintness, double vision and confusion (Table 8.1). Loss of balance, together with awkward, irritable or aggressive behaviour, may lead to arrest by the police for being drunk and disorderly.

Table 8.1 Distinguishing features of hyperglycaemia and hypoglycaemia (insulin shock)

Feature	*HYPERglycaemia*	*HYPOglycaemia*
Onset	gradual	sudden
Food intake	normal	reduced
Preceding illness or stress	yes	no
Acetone smell on breath	yes	no
Skin	dry and flushed	moist and pale
Respiration	air-hunger	normal
Pulse	weak and rapid	strong and bounding
Thirst	yes	no

The low blood sugar leads to a secretion of adrenaline, which produces a pale, sweating skin and an increase in the pulse rate.

Eventually the casualty becomes unconscious, because the brain needs a certain level of sugar to maintain its function.

HYPERGLYCAEMIA

This is caused by carelessness in omitting insulin, or by an acute infection together with failure to increase the dose of insulin while the infection is present.

The slow rise in blood sugar produces a slow onset of symptoms (Table 8.1). Glucose is excreted in the urine, together with large quantities of urine (polyuria). If the condition remains undetected for a long time, there may be a severe loss of water from the body, producing thirst and dehydration. Vomiting and abdominal pain may also occur.

As the body is unable to use the available glucose, a sense of fatigue develops. Body fats are metabolized to provide energy and acetone is produced, giving a characteristic smell to the breath. The blood becomes slightly more acidic and this stimulates the respiratory centre to increase the rate of respiration (air-hunger).

The continued rise in the blood sugar increases the severity of the symptoms and the casualty becomes unconscious.

FIRST-AID MANAGEMENT OF THE DIABETIC EMERGENCY

The diabetic emergency most likely to be encountered is hypoglycaemia. This can be corrected quite easily if recognized early, and the diabetic patient should learn to recognize the symptoms. The frequent cause is a lack of glucose and the first-aid management of hypoglycaemia is simply to give sugar. Diabetics should carry an emergency supply of glucose in the form of sweets or sugar lumps.

This method of treatment may be thwarted if the casualty is unconscious and therefore unable to swallow. No attempt must be made to force sweet drinks down the throat. The casualty should be placed in the recovery position and sent to hospital.

In some cases there may be difficulty in deciding whether the casualty is suffering from hypoglycaemia or hyperglycaemia. He may be in a confused state – unable to give any information regarding his intake of insulin or food. Under these circumstances the first-aider must give some form of glucose, if the casualty is able to swallow. If the casualty is suffering from hypoglycaemia, the intake of glucose will result in a speedy recovery. If hyperglycaemia is present the anticipated recovery will not take place. However, the small amount of added glucose will not harm the casualty, who should be placed in the recovery position and transported urgently to hospital.

9 Miscellaneous

THE EFFECTS OF TEMPERATURE ON THE BODY

The body's temperature is controlled by the temperature regulating centre in the brain. A small amount of heat is produced by basic metabolism and muscle activity. The temperature regulating centre can control the temperature by:

(1) Altering the skin circulation. Dilating the blood vessels in the skin increases the blood flow through the skin and increases the heat loss. The casualty has a hot, flushed appearance. Constricting the blood vessels reduces the flow of blood and heat is conserved.

(2) Producing sweat from the skin's sweat glands. A surface loses far more heat when it is wet. However, if the humidity of the air is high, the sweat does not evaporate quickly enough and heat loss is reduced.

Loss of control of body temperature may result in fever, hyperthermia or hypothermia.

Fever – the body temperature is above 37.0 °C (98.6 °F)
Hyperthermia – the body temperature is above 40.5 °C (105 °F)
Hypothermia – the body temperature is below 35.0 °C (90 °F)

Excessive heat may produce:

(1) heat exhaustion,
(2) heat stroke.

Heat exhaustion

This develops over a few days when the casualty fails to become acclimatized to the heat and is caused by the body becoming depleted of salt and water. The casualty complains of fatigue, giddiness, headache, irritability and muscle cramps. The casualty gives the appearance of shock, with profuse sweating, but the body temperature is normal.

The casualty should be removed to a cooler place and an attempt made, if the casualty is conscious, to replace the lost salt and fluids. Half a teaspoon of salt in 500 ml of water should improve the casualty's condition. The indiscriminate intake of salt tablets without an adequate intake of water must be avoided, as this is certain to upset the body chemistry, by drawing fluid out of the tissues.

Heat stroke

This is produced by prolonged exposure to high temperatures in the environment, or illness – such as pneumonia, meningitis or malaria. The heat regulating mechanism fails and temperatures of 40.5 °C (105 °F) or more may be produced.

The casualty becomes irritable and complains of a headache and dizziness. The pulse increases to 140–160 per minute. Unconsciousness may develop rapidly, leading to convulsions and death.

The condition must be regarded as a medical emergency and medical aid requested immediately. The aim of treatment is to reduce the casualty's temperature as quickly as possible, until it reaches a normal level. His clothing should be removed and if he is unconscious he should be placed in the recovery position. The body surface is kept moist by sponging or using sprays of water, and fans are used to direct cool air towards the casualty, encouraging evaporation.

When the temperature has returned to normal, the casualty can be dried, covered with a dry sheet and placed in a cool room to await medical aid.

Excessive cold may produce:

(1) Exposure
(2) Hypothermia

Exposure

Problems caused by exposure are usually encountered when the ill-prepared go hill walking in poor weather conditions. Of course, problems can also occur when well prepared walkers are caught by an unexpected change in the weather. The problems are aggravated by an increase in heat loss from wet clothing and cold winds, and when the casualty is exhausted and hungry.

Lowering the body temperature slows the functions of the body. The casualty may be unable to keep up with his companions. He is unable to answer questions coherently and becomes unconscious with a slow, irregular heartbeat and a slow respiration rate.

Treatment is aimed at preventing any further loss of heat by providing the casualty with shelter and exchanging the wet clothing for dry. High calorie foods and warm drinks will help to improve the body temperature.

A particularly dangerous situation occurs when a person is suffering from the effects of excessive alcohol consumption and is staggering home in very cold weather. The effect of the alcohol is to dilate the blood vessels in the skin – thereby increasing the heat loss. The problem is intensified if he falls into snow and remains unconscious from the effects of the alcohol.

Hypothermia

Hypothermia exists when the body's core temperature falls below 35 °C and can affect both infants and the elderly. They may both experience difficulty in controlling their body temperature, which may fall to 25 °C (77 °F). If the temperature falls below this level, the chances of recovery are slim.

The *infant* may look quite fit and healthy, with a pink colour – but is also drowsy, listless and refusing feeds.

The *elderly* are at risk during the winter months, when they may spend several days alone in a cold house. Because of poor weather and poor mobility, they are unable to get to the shops to get food.

Their meals become inadequate and they begin to lose interest in normal daily living. Despite wrapping themselves in several layers of clothing, they still lose heat faster than they can generate it – and they slip into hypothermia.

The person becomes confused and drowsy with a slow respiration and pulse, and he feels very cold.

Treatment involves simply removing the casualty from the cold environment into a warm room. Several layers of warm clothing can be used to gradually re-warm the casualty. Rapid warming must be avoided because this would produce an increased blood flow through the skin, resulting in further heat loss. For the same reason, alcohol must not be given to the casualty. Well-padded hot water bottles can be applied to the trunk area, but not to the limbs. Transferring the casualty to a warm hospital ward is usually sufficient treatment to overcome hypothermia.

The chances of recovery are less when the casualty is very old, frail and suffering from a co-existing disease, such as diabetes or pneumonia.

CRUSH INJURY

The crush syndrome occurs when limbs have suffered extensive and prolonged crushing. The crushing of a small area of the body, for example the hand, important though it is, is not included in the crush syndrome. As a result of the crushing injury, the blood vessels involved become damaged and leak plasma into the surrounding tissues. The limb will therefore become swollen and it may become numb and tingle. As a result of leaking plasma, the circulating blood volume drops and the casualty becomes severely shocked. When the crushed limb is released the leakage of plasma continues and the blood pressure may fall quite alarmingly. As well as increasing the shock it has a harmful effect on the kidneys, and this may lead to renal failure and death. Toxins are released from the damaged muscles and these can also produce kidney damage.

Where the casualty has been crushed for more than 30 minutes the first-aider should summon the emergency services before attempting to release the casualty. The Medical Flying Squad may also be required to give intravenous pain-relieving drugs, and in some cases the affected limb may have to be amputated. Apart from the basic first-aid management of controlling haemorrhage, dealing with fractures, and controlling shock, it is most important to record the length of time the limb has been crushed and also the time that the limb was released. If the affected limb has not been fractured, it is better to elevate it, in an attempt to counteract any further leakage of plasma from the circulation. Respiration and heart rate should be checked at frequent intervals as resuscitation may be required. It is important that everyone who is involved in direct care of the casualty should be aware that he has suffered a crush injury.

TETANUS

Tetanus is caused by a spore-bearing bacterium, *Clostridium tetani*. The spores can occur anywhere, but are very likely to be encountered in the soil in agricultural areas, as they are found in the faeces of cows and horses. The spores can exist almost indefinitely. Once they have gained access to the body through a wound contaminated by soil, the spores germinate and produce a very powerful toxin, tetanospasmin, which affects the central nervous system, producing muscle rigidity and spasm. The tetanus bacillus multiplies best in deep wounds where air is in short supply or absent – as in puncture wounds caused by a garden fork.

The first symptom is usually trismus or lockjaw – a painful spasm of the jaw muscles producing difficulty in opening the mouth. Any muscle can be involved and if the muscles of respiration are affected, respiratory distress will be produced. The muscle spasm may be triggered by noise or coughing.

Management

All wounds should be regarded as potential points of entry for tetanus spores and, at the time of injury, as much foreign material as possible should be removed from the wound. If the circumstances indicate that there is a potential risk of tetanus, the casualty should be advised to seek urgent medical advice regarding tetanus toxoid, or tetanus immunoglobulin for more immediate protection.

The time between the injury and the onset of tetanus is 5–15 days. The mortality is quite high, with about 20% of people who contract tetanus dying from the disease.

The principal preventive procedure is active immunization. An attack of tetanus does not give any immunity. The routine programme of immunization in children offers some protection to the individual, but the protection needs enhancing with a booster injection every 5–10 years. Many wounds that cause tetanus are relatively minor and no first aid or medical treatment is sought – emphasizing the importance of immunization. People who are more at risk from contracting tetanus, such as gardeners and farm-workers, should be reminded of the need to maintain adequate protection with immunization.

RABIES

Rabies is caused by a virus which is transmitted to man by the bite of a rabies-infected animal. The virus attacks the central nervous system and usually causes death.

In Europe, rabies is carried by dogs, foxes and wolves. Although the incidence of rabies in foxes is higher (80% of all affected animals are foxes), the majority of cases of human rabies are caused by bites from dogs – indicating the closer relationship man has with dogs.

Import controls and quarantine regulations are effective methods of preventing the introduction of the disease into the country. The few cases of rabies that have occurred have resulted from bites sustained while abroad.

A bite or lick from a rabid animal inoculates the saliva, loaded with virus, through the skin. People travelling to countries where rabies is prevalent should avoid unnecessary contact with wild or stray animals.

Management

If a person is bitten by a suspected rabid animal, the wound should be scrubbed with soap and water under a running tap for about 5 minutes. The area should then be rinsed with water. If the owner of the animal can be contacted, advice should be sought regarding the immunization status of the animal. Local medical advice should be sought rather than waiting to return home before seeking advice.

The incubation period varies between 3 weeks and 3 months and the shortest time occurs if a child is bitten on the face.

Symptoms include headache, dry mouth, thirst, restlessness and excitability. The presence of a dry mouth and thirst lead to a desire for water to drink. However, the sight or sound of water produces an intense fear of drinking (hydrophobia) resulting in increased excitability, with the casualty becoming wild and hallucinating. Convulsions and coma occur.

Treatment with injections should be started as soon as possible after the bite, to try and neutralize the virus before it can affect the central nervous system.

THE MANAGEMENT OF PSYCHIATRIC EMERGENCIES

Psychiatric illness will only rarely require help from a first-aider – either when the psychiatric illness commences as an acute emergency or when the long-term control of an illness becomes unstable.

Depending on the circumstances, the first-aider should be sympathetic and friendly, seeking to calm and reassure the patient. The patient may be suffering from an illness which may make him become unexpectedly aggressive and violent – and the first-aider should be aware of this possibility at all times. If the patient is thought to be a source of danger to himself or others, the first-aider should consider sending for the police. If the psychiatric illness has been present for a long time, he may already be under treatment and supervision. In that case he may be known to the Social Services Department and the Duty Social Worker should be involved. The patient cannot be admitted to a Psychiatric Hospital against his will unless certain medico-legal manoeuvres are carried out by the doctor and the social worker.

The aim of the first-aider must be to provide support in the acute situation whilst medical help is obtained. There is no need to waste time attempting to arrive at a psychiatric diagnosis – and there is no place for the amateur psychiatrist in the field of first aid.

Anxiety state

A mild anxiety state is fairly common for most people and can be said to result from the stresses of life. It can be brought on by fear, reaction to unexpected news or an anxious anticipation of an event. In its mild form it can be regarded as giving some protection to the individual, by making him aware of imminent danger and preparing him, in both physical and psychological terms, to cope with that danger either by fright or flight. Most people manage to cope with their episodes of mild anxiety and the first-aider is unlikely to be asked for help.

It is often difficult to draw the line between a normal anxiety reaction and an acute anxiety state. It depends on the circumstances and the reaction the individual has to a certain level of stress. Some people can cope quite adequately with a level of stress that other people would find quite intolerable.

When the anxiety is related to a specific object or activity (cats, mice, travelling in buses, etc.) it is called a phobic anxiety state, or phobia.

Clinical features of anxiety

If the level of anxiety increases, the patient may develop symptoms of pallor, dry mouth, sweating, dizziness, frequency of micturition and an increased pulse rate. The respiration rate may increase, leading to the hyperventilation syndrome – increasing faintness, a feeling of pins and needles in the limbs, and spasm of the muscles of the forearm and hand.

First-aid management of anxiety

An attempt should be made to discover what provoked the episode of anxiety. Reassurance may be all that is required to calm the patient down, but if the episode continues, medical help should be requested.

Hysteria

Hysteria can affect people in several ways, but the conditions most likely to be encountered are:

(1) simple hysteria,
(2) hysterical disorders (conversion hysteria).

Simple hysteria

In popular usage, hysteria describes the state of mind when a person goes 'out of control' and behaves in an exaggerated, embarrassing manner. There is usually a 'trigger' event, which most people would regard as a horrifying one, but situations of mild stress may produce a similar state.

The symptoms and signs can be numerous and varied, but the most dramatic involve shaking, shouting and screaming, abnormal posture and wild movements of the arms and legs. There may be some resemblance to an epileptic fit, but hysteria can usually be distinguished from epilepsy by the absence of incontinence, an increase in the exaggerated movements if gentle restraint is attempted, and the absence of cyanosis. Respiration may increase and result in the hyperventilation syndrome with symptoms of increasing faintness, a feeling of pins and needles in the limbs, and spasm of the muscles of the forearm and hand.

Occasionally mass hysteria may be encountered, most commonly in girls' schools, where, under certain circumstances, there is an apparent epidemic of sudden fainting attacks, vomiting or abdominal pain.

Hysterical disorders (conversion hysteria)

In this form of hysteria the person complains of something which mimics a physical illness, such as a loss of sensation in one part of the body, paralysis of one or more limbs, or blindness. This is usually the result of stress in a susceptible person – but can occur in normal individuals at a time of overwhelming stress (war or mass casualties at a disaster).

Diagnosis and management of hysteria

The diagnosis of hysteria can be very difficult when the symptoms mimic a physical illness – and easier when the stressful situation is apparent and the symptoms relate to exaggerated and bizarre behaviour.

Intense reassurance and support is required while medical help is obtained.

Depression

A *depressed mood,* resembling sadness or grief, is a state which everyone experiences from time to time. It usually occurs in response to the disappointments and frustrations of life – but can occur for no apparent reason.

A persistent depressed mood results in a *depressive illness.* Symptoms of insomnia, loss of appetite and weight loss occur; the world seems dark, the future looks bleak and there seems no point in living.

Depression can occur shortly after childbirth and is then called *puerperal depression.* Feelings of inadequacy and a general inability to cope with the baby are coupled with lack of sleep from disturbed nights attending to the baby. An acute depression may be associated with a resentment of the baby and little desire to look after the baby, other members of the family, or herself.

Suicide

Acute depression may lead to suicide and the first-aider should be aware of this possibility when dealing with a depressed person. Threats of suicide should never be ignored, especially if there has been a previous suicide attempt, a family history of suicide or preoccupation with talk of suicide. Physical illness (cancer and the fear of it) is present in a high proportion of elderly people who commit suicide.

In the absence of any definite physical or mental illness an attempt at suicide is often regarded as a 'gesture' or a 'cry for help' in response to an intolerable situation at home or at work. The act may succeed if the plan is miscalculated and resuscitation is not forthcoming. 20% of suicides leave a note indicating premeditation, and this often contains ideas of guilt or despair.

Management of a suicide threat

If a person announces that he is going to commit suicide, the desire to die is often temporary. The person is facing an immediate crisis and should be reassured that the crisis can be resolved.

(1) Communicate with him to establish a relationship.
(2) Help him to identify the cause of the crisis.

(3) Offer constructive help towards resolving the crisis.
(4) Involve the patient's family and friends to remind him that other people care for him.
(5) Depending on the circumstances, advise him to consult his doctor, or stay with him until medical help is obtained.

Schizophrenia

Although schizophrenia means 'split mind' it was not intended to mean split personality or split into two parts. The condition produces a fragmentation of ideas and emotion. It usually starts in early adult life and results in odd ways of thinking and behaving.

The patient may feel that his thoughts are being controlled, and ideas put into his mind. He may believe that comments on the radio or in the newspaper are about him. Hallucinations may occur in the form of 'voices' talking to him and giving him instructions.

The first-aider may be involved when there is an acute behavioural disturbance. Episodes of wild excitement and impulsive behaviour may occur. There is also a risk of a violent outburst or a serious and senseless criminal act being committed.

At the acute stage the schizophrenic may need to be admitted to hospital to protect himself and others.

Glossary

Acetabulum	The socket of the hip joint, where the femur to joins the hip bone
Air-hunger	Increased rate and depth of breathing
Anaphylactic	Generalized allergic reaction producing a life-threatening situation
Antidote	Substance which neutralizes the harmful effects of a specific poison
Asphyxia	Lack of oxygen in the blood
Automatism	State of behaving automatically, without being aware of surroundings or events
Callus	Immature bone laid down at a fracture during the healing process
Cardiogenic	Arising from, or related to, the heart
Cyanosis	Blueness of the lips, finger-ends and ear-lobes
Dermis	Layer of skin under the epidermis
Dilate	Enlarge
Epidermis	Top layer of skin
Exudate	Fluid that leaks from the surface of a wound in response to infection or burn
Grand mal	Form of epilepsy producing characteristic convulsive movements
Granulation tissue	Cells which actively grow to produce healing tissue at a wound
Haematoma	Collection of blood
Hydrophobia	Fear of water
Hyperglycaemia	High level of blood sugar

Hyperthermia	Body temperature above 40.5 °C (105 °F)
Hypoglycaemia	Low level of blood sugar
Hypothermia	Body temperature below 35 °C (90 °F)
Hypovolaemia	Reduced blood volume – from loss of fluid
Immunization	Prevention of infection by helping the body develop its own protection
Inflammation	The response of living tissue to injury from trauma, heat, infection or chemicals
Intravenous	Injected directly into a vein
Neurogenic	Arising from, or related to, the brain or nerve supply to the body
Petit mal	Form of epilepsy without characteristic convulsive movements
Polyuria	Production of excessive amounts of urine
Pulmonary circulation	Part of the circulatory system taking blood from the heart to the lungs and back again
Septicaemia	Infection of the bloodstream
Septum	Dividing 'wall' of tissue
Subcutaneous	Immediately under the dermis
Systemic circulation	Part of the circulatory system taking blood from the heart to the rest of the body, excluding the lungs, and back again
Thrombus	Blood clot in a blood vessel
Toxin	Harmful substance which may damage the body

Index

GPSR Compliance

The European Union's (EU) General Product Safety Regulation (GPSR) is a set of rules that requires consumer products to be safe and our obligations to ensure this.

If you have any concerns about our products, you can contact us on ProductSafety@springernature.com

In case Publisher is established outside the EU, the EU authorized representative is:

Springer Nature Customer Service Center GmbH
Europaplatz 3
69115 Heidelberg, Germany

Batch number: 10830935

Printed by Printforce, the Netherlands